By Richard Watson

THE DOWNFALL OF CARTESIANISM

MAN AND NATURE (with Patty Jo Watson)

THE LONGEST CAVE (with Roger W. Brucker)

UNDER PLOWMAN'S FLOOR (a novel)

THE RUNNER (a novel)

THE PHILOSOPHER'S DIET

THE
PHILOSOPHER'S
DIET

THE PHILOSOPHER'S DIET

How to Lose Weight and Change the World

Richard Watson

The Atlantic Monthly Press
BOSTON / NEW YORK

FIRST EDITION

Chapter seven appeared, in
slightly different form, in
The Georgia Review.

LIBRARY OF CONGRESS CATALOGING IN PUBLICATION DATA

Watson, Richard A., 1931–
The philosopher's diet.

1. Reducing diets. 2. Health. I. Title.
RM222.2.W277 1985   613.2′5   84-45818
ISBN 0-87113-016-5

BP

Published simultaneously in Canada

PRINTED IN THE UNITED STATES OF AMERICA

War came.
Bodies lined the roadside.
Their fat sizzled in the sun.
> — *Lamentation for the Destruction of Ur*
> Third Millennium B.C.

Diet. . . . Course of life: way of living or
thinking. . . . To regulate oneself.
> — *Oxford English Dictionary*

Cautionary Note

The author urgently recommends that before you act on the advice in this book, you have a thorough medical examination and get your doctor's approval of the program. This probably is not necessary for normally healthy adults, but who knows from normal? I don't want to get sued.

Acknowledgments

The Philosopher's Diet was written while I was engaged in Cartesian studies at the Center for Advanced Study in the Behavioral Sciences, Stanford, California. I thank Center Director Gardner Lindzey and the Board of Trustees for their indulgence and understanding. As Descartes said, give a man leisure and truth will out.

I want also to thank the Center Fellows and staff for encouragement and inspiration, particularly Carol Smith for laying on the last straw. Others to whom I am indebted are legion, but many of them are mentioned in the text. One who is not is Peter Davison, an editor of rare acumen. I thank them one and all.

Contents

THE
PHILOSOPHER'S
DIET

Introduction

IN this book I tell how to take off weight and keep it off. The book also embodies a philosophy of life. The weight program is the content of the book, the philosophy of life is its form.

I take it for granted that you have asked yourself in these trying times what it all means. What does it all mean? And why don't philosophers tell us? A few years ago my mother asked me these two questions. She was seventy, her children were grown and gone from home, and she and my father had nothing to do but tend their garden, read, and watch television. She had a son who was a professional philosopher. She wanted to know. Why wouldn't I tell her?

My mother is not alone in her indignation. The editors of *Time* also would like to know what it all means. The editors of the *Atlantic Monthly*, of the *Partisan Review*, of the *New York Times* — they would like to know, too. Hugh Hefner, editor of *Playboy*, got so dissatisfied with the professionals a few years ago that he decided to have a go at it himself. Not only that, he sent copies of his work to many of us philosophers to set us straight. He wrote twenty-two installments of "The Playboy Philosophy" before he came to a stop. I have a chapter titled "Sex" myself.

For, as you have discerned, I have decided to take the complaints seriously. Why *don't* philosophers tell you what it all means? The answer is simple. They don't know. And I don't know much more than the others, but it just happens that I do know a number of things that, as Descartes said, it would be shameful of me to withhold. So I wrote a book.

Before you read this book, you doubtless want to know what my philosophy is. And in two sentences. Very well, let me say that I find these to be peculiar times. Some of us live the most extraordinarily satisfying lives in a century that has witnessed the genocidal slaughter of six million Jews; a world in which atom bombs have been dropped on Japanese cities, in which torture is common, and in which hundreds of millions of people live in conditions of abject poverty, starvation, oppression, and hopelessness. The leaders of Russia and the United States seem determined to go to war with one another sooner or later, and they have enough nerve gas and germs (never mind the panoply of nuclear, hydrogen, and neutron bombs) to wipe us all out. My daughter, who is twenty, thinks someone will push the button, and she asks me what we can do about it. I don't know. Probably nothing. My wife, who is an archeologist, says there have always been winners and losers. Some of the earliest written records are about atrocities of war. For example, the key text for cracking the cuneiform code is a description of what Darius did to rebels in the fourth century B.C. He cut off their ears, put out their eyes, cut off their noses, and then dragged them behind his chariots in chains.

But you wanted to know my philosophy. It has to do with reading (covered in the chapter on "How to Live") and writing (covered in the chapter on "How to Die"). This philosophy is derived primarily from my Welsh mother and my Scots father. When I was very young, my mother used to sit beside me to make me practice the piano. "Let's get on with it," she would say. My father also had a saying. When I sought sympathy after stubbing a toe or falling down and skinning my knee, he would say, "Rub dirt in it." Two sentences.

So let's get on with it.

1
Fat

Fat. I presume you want to get rid of it. Then quit eating so much. No normally healthy person on the good green earth ever got thinner without cutting down on caloric intake. Do a few exercises, don't eat so much, and you will lose weight.

Ah, but it's not so easy. Else why would there be such a market for diet books? The reason is a secret I intend to tell.

There are a lot of good things about fat. For one thing, it tastes good, especially in ice cream or dripping from hot barbecued ribs. More important, you could not live without it. Your body is working all the time, heart beating, blood circulating, lungs breathing, and unless you eat all the time, fuel must be stored to keep the body working. Fat is fuel. Human bodies are superb organisms for storing fat, presumably because our ancestors evolved through times of feast and famine. There is nothing wrong with having a little store of fat right now. When you read in the newspaper about people marooned in Alaska by an airplane crash, you find that the fat ones survive. And it is always good to have some fat in excess in case you get sick and lose weight. Once the fat goes, your body starts eating up your muscles and organs, and then you are really in trouble. Fat helps keep you warm, too, in case the airplane crashes in cold water. Skinny people starve and freeze a lot sooner than fat people. That's why many Americans who lived through the Depression and Germans who lived through World War II are fat today: they don't trust tomorrow. As for today, there is a lot of unemployment, and it could happen to you. My brother-in-law, who is an ex-air-traffic controller, particularly advises anyone who intends to strike against the government to fatten up first.

So what are diet books for? They provide light reading for moderately heavy people. Just reading a diet book relieves some anxiety about one's weight. This is because most people who buy diet books aren't really fat. They fret about it a lot, but these diet groupies are seldom more than 20 or 30 pounds over the average healthy weight recommended by doctors and federal agencies. Suppose you are a man who "ought" to weigh 150, but you weigh 175. Or a woman who "ought" to weigh 110 but weighs 130. You may look pudgy in comparison with fashion models, but you can carry it. Listen, the government gives you some leeway when it comes to fat. The Feds set a standard, but you have to be *fat* to get turned down by the Army. Consider someone with high standards. The painter Peter Paul

Rubens would not have looked twice at most of today's self-designated overweight women. And he did not love fat women: his models were voluptuous. A lot of us have a thing about voluptuous women. They have always done all right, they are doing all right, they always will do all right.

Really fat people seldom buy diet books and seldom go on diets. Some of them are not very healthy, some of them have quite serious problems, and some of them don't care. Not one in a thousand of the obese thinks a diet book will help, so they don't bother. Still, there are always exceptions, and my book could be for one of them, too.

Let's get back to your average "overweight" American. People usually fret about fat because of vanity. Deep down, of course, most of us know that we will never look like a fashion model. We aren't built that way, we can't afford that kind of clothing or wouldn't wear such a bathing suit. We know it would be a lot of trouble, even if we were, could, or would. On top of all that, we keep growing older. Still, we can dream that we look like the beautiful ones. Just going on a diet makes you feel better about your looks, and there is the added pleasure of boring your friends by talking about your diet.

The diet industry (philosophical analysis reveals) is part of the entertainment business. It belongs to the specialized branch that manufactures unnecessary things to do. Going on a diet is like playing solitaire. But unlike playing solitaire, dieting is approved by most people as an activity requiring moral fiber. To attain this preferred status, start a diet and (most important) tell people you have. You can talk self-righteously about dieting in any company. Almost nobody takes off a lot of fat and keeps it off. If they do, serious dieters ostracize them. The only socially acceptable thin dieters are those who write the diet books, although you will find that they have few fat friends.

Dieting is a serious business, but most dieters are not serious about maintaining the weight they reach after they've taken off a few pounds. They gain them back, and then lose them again. "Oh, here I go again," they say.

What if you do want to take the fat off and keep it off? That's an interesting question. So is the answer, but it will take a while. Hang on.

Let's start like a philosopher, with another question. Are many Americans as overweight as they think they are? Consider a government formula for determining the average weight of American adults who range from about 5′0″ to 6′4″ tall. For men, you count 110 pounds for the first 5 feet and add 5½ pounds for each inch above 5 feet. For women, you count 100 pounds for the first 5 feet and add 5 pounds for each inch above 5 feet. Thus, the average weight of an American woman 5′3″ tall is 115 pounds. This is dry, nude weight. Weights more or less on this order are "right" for normal healthy people. A lot of people fit in that range. (Where do you think they got the average in the first place? By weighing a lot of Americans, adding up all their weights, and averaging them out.)

There are many healthy men 5′8″ tall who weigh anywhere between 134 and 174 pounds. What if you dressed them all in three-piece suits? They would all look much the same unless you stood a pair of the extremes side by side. If you check in at the average weight, do you get a prize? No, all the weights in this 40-pound range are normal.

Indeed, there is no reason why the average should even be healthy. Dr. George Sheehan (who writes a column for *Runner's World*) claims that the healthiest weight is 10 percent below the average. Thus, the healthiest 5′8″ male (all other things being equal) would weigh 138.6 pounds, and the healthiest 5′3″ female, 103.5 pounds. That's where the squeeze begins. Suppose you are a perfectly comfortable 5′8″ male weighing in at 174 pounds. If you want to be at the national average, you must lose 20 pounds. But if you want to be healthiest according to Dr. Sheehan, you've got to lose 30.8 pounds.

You need not stop there. Dr. Ernst van Aaken (who used to write a column for *Runner's World*) says the best running weight is 20 percent off the average. So a 5′3″ woman weighing 130 pounds, though perfectly within the normal average range, would have to lose 15 pounds to match the abstract American average, 26.5 pounds to be healthy according to Dr. Sheehan, and 38 pounds to run for Dr. Van Aaken.

I know people who have the magic weights, but almost none of them dieted to get there. In fact, most of those who fall below the American average are trying to gain weight to reach it.

If this is beginning to seem pretty silly, that's just the point. Because you don't fit the government's figure for average weight exactly does not mean that you should fret about fat and dieting or that you are over-weight or unhealthy. The average figure is simply an abstract measurement and has no necessary connection whatever with health or being overweight. If everyone were really unhealthily overweight, then the average would be unhealthy. As it turns out, the American average is perfectly healthy according to most of the medical profession. If you want to get down to Dr. Sheehan's figure, fine, it probably won't hurt you. Unless you want to be a world-class runner, however, or you just naturally weigh very little, stay away from Dr. Van Aaken. Furthermore, if you do have to lose weight because of a heart problem, diabetes, or what-ever, your doctor will either scare the dickens out of you so you stay on your diet, or he won't and you might die. I would stick to my diet if my doctor told me I would pop off otherwise.

Now does all this rather ridiculous fretting about your weight do you any harm? Nah. Or, let's put it this way: if you have anorexia nervosa you might starve yourself to death, and if you have bulimia you might eat yourself to death. If you are not sick, fretting about your weight is probably better for you than fretting about something you can't do anything about, such as whether or not the President will push a button and start the nuclear holocaust.

My sister, who is a radicalized housewife and "part-time" employee in one of America's major service industries ("part-time" in quotes because although she works full-time, they won't designate her as such, for then they'd have to pay benefits), points out to me that being overweight in America has nothing to do with health, but everything to do with fads and fashions. Women who are much above or even at the average figure are perceived as being overweight. This perception, usually more by other women than by men, is what is important. You might conclude that if you don't want to be seen as a fat slob, then diet. I'm opposed to this kind of argument. You shouldn't diet just because the clothing industry hires emaciated models. Let's try to rise above that kind of pressure.

Still, I know that it doesn't help to be told that Polynesians and Turks and Peter Paul Rubens love fat women. Or that Lillian Russell, the toast of the 1890s, weighed 200 pounds and was thought to be a sylph. Today, you don't have to be as thin as Twiggy or David Bowie to get admiring comments from your friends. All you have to do is stay on the low side of Margaret Rutherford and Marlon Brando.

You could just wait. Styles are bound to change, but what about all that subtle peer pressure that is so pervasive now, however faddish? Well, all right, there is a way. You can lose weight and keep it off if you want to do the necessary work.

It is very hard to do, but it won't hurt you (or anyone else). In the long run it probably will be healthy for you — if you succeed and stick with it, that is. Don't keep gaining and losing a lot of weight over and over; that's not good for you. So stay up or down, one or the other. You want to go down? Right.

I don't want to bother with you unless you are serious about losing at least 20 pounds. If you want to lose 30, it will be even more fun. If you want to shed even more, I might get you down, but it would be awfully hard to keep you there. Let's be reasonable. Suppose you're a woman 5′3″ tall, weighing in at 130 pounds, and you want to weigh 110 pounds. One hundred and ten pounds forever! Let's do it. (If you are a man, make the necessary changes in the example, *mutatis mutandis*, as we philosophers say.)

How? Without mincing words: eat less. But that alone is not enough, for you also have to learn how to eat differently from the way you are eating now so you can stay at 110 when you get there. You must modify your eating behavior. You begin by reading inspirational literature. I'll provide my share in these pages, but I can't begin to provide enough. So the first thing you must do is go out to buy or borrow some books on dieting, calories, fat, salt, fiber, sugar, exercise, fasting, and natural foods. It does not matter which books you get — go for quantity, not quality.

And *do go out*. As you'll see, leaving the kitchen for exercise is part of the program. Lots of books. Put some in the bathroom, some by your bed, some in the kitchen, and a couple in your briefcase or backpack or purse, and some in your desk at home and some in your desk at work. You will read these books over and over again. It feels good to read them, even when you are off your diet. Inspirational literature assures you that somebody cares, that there is a way, and that you can be saved.

Ready? Now you must face the primary truth of dieting. Losing weight means cutting down on the food you eat. Across the board. Food fad diets lead neither to health nor to permanent weight loss. Those nutty diets are fun to read about, and some of the craziest books are the best inspirational reading, but you certainly cannot live the rest of your life on grapefruit or steak. People who take weight off with crank diets may be highly visible dieters, that is, they do a lot of dieting in public, but they are not serious about taking weight off and keeping it off. To do that, you have to establish a balanced diet that you can maintain after you reach your desired weight. You can find out about the normal healthy balance of foods by reading almost any book on health and nutrition. I'm just going to assume that you know. Then you cut down, keeping the healthy nutritional balance, until you start to lose weight. I know you are in a hurry, so let's start with a 900-calorie diet. That's 900 calories a day, and it isn't much.

Memorize the figures in one of your calorie counters

(you need a couple of them, of course). This is not hard to do because you can lump the foods in categories and fairly soon learn that a large apple or orange or a medium banana is about 100 calories, most cheeses are about 100 calories an ounce, and so on. Just take your normal balanced diet and cut it down to 900 calories. You can look in any number of books that provide balanced 900-calorie diets of normal food. Step one is to get on a 900-calorie diet and stick to it.

Parenthetically, let me now give a crucial instruction. Always count your calories. You will soon learn to keep track in your head, but if you tend to cheat unconsciously, write them down. You might as well get used to counting calories, because you will probably have to do it *the rest of your life*. Calories are additive from day to day, so if you eat 100 too many one day, cut off 100 the next day. Does that mean that if you fast for two days on a 900-calorie diet, you can gorge on 2700 calories the third day? I suppose, but that is not exactly what philosophers mean by either a balanced diet or a balanced life.

It may take a long time for you to reach your desired weight, but when you do, here is step two. Go to a 1500-calorie diet. Try it for a week. If you continue to lose, increase it to 1800. You may have to juggle it back and forth, but at 5'3" for a woman, trying to hold firm, you might reach a maintenance diet of between 1800 and 2200 calories. For a 5'8" man, it might be between 2200 and 2400 calories.

After you establish a maintenance diet for your desired weight, you are ready for permanent step three.

You must always eat your maintenance diet to stay at your desired weight. Eating exactly the right amount to stay trim may be something rats and raccoons in the wild do instinctively, but we humans are domesticated animals, like pigs, and most of us will eat whatever is put in the trough until it's gone. You must continue to count the calories. Cut down on the morrow what you over-ate the day before. Keeping the faith is keeping count.

Not so easy?

I agree. The program I've outlined is too reasonable to be easy. It isn't radical enough. What's more, it won't work.

It won't work because you are still eating all the stuff you like, the sort of food you have always eaten. Once you get down to your desired weight and ease off, you will start eating more and more of the same old things again, and whammo! you will soon be bloated again. It isn't radical enough to work because it does not change your eating habits in the right way. To lower your weight 20 pounds or more and keep that lower weight is to change your life. Anyone can go on a diet. Let's make a real *change*.

What tastes best? What do we all crave? Sugar. During the last 100 years or so, the average American went from consuming about 12 pounds of processed sugar a year to consuming over 100 pounds a year.

Because it was there. A healthy person needs absolutely none of that processed sugar. So cut it out. In effect, you must avoid almost all processed foods — foods that come sealed in bags, boxes, packages, cans, bottles, and jars. You think I'm kidding, don't you? Believe me, I know what I'm talking about. If you follow my advice you will eat better in two senses: first, fresh food is better for you, and second, it tastes better than processed foods. Here is why.

Foods are processed so they can be preserved for storage and shipment. Although some of the chemicals used as preservatives may eventually cause cancer, so does the polluted air you breathe, and I'm not going to get off on that subject. The main problem with processed foods is that they contain enormous quantities of salt and sugar. These are added as preservatives and taste-enhancers. Also, meat, fruit, and vegetables on the verge of spoiling can be made quite palatable with salt and sugar. Salt makes you want to eat and drink more. Sugar is addicting. It is perfectly intelligent marketing practice, then, for manufacturers to shoot processed foods full of salt and sugar (and if both are put in at the same time, they counteract each other so even more can be put in). Is it surprising that manufacturers want you to eat more of their foodstuffs? Another addicting additive is caffeine. Add eight teaspoons of sugar, some flavor, and a bit of caffeine to eight ounces of carbonated water, and you have one of the best-selling drinks in the world. At least knock off the sugar. If you need the caffeine, drink coffee, black. If you still crave the carbonation, you'd best go to seltzer water. From what I can make of all the reports, the artificial flavors, colorings, and sweetenings in diet drinks may be more harmful in the long run than the sugar-loaded originals.

You *need* the sugar? There is plenty of sugar in fresh fruits and vegetables, and the carbohydrates in grains are easily converted to sugar by digestion. Two medium-sized apples have about the same amount of sugar as a bottle of soda pop. And besides giving you lots of vitamins and minerals and roughage, two apples will probably cut down your total consumption in a way a bottle of soda pop will not.

The worst processed food is, of course, sugar itself. Your body turns excess sugar into fat. Does eating a lot of sugar cause hypoglycemia or diabetes? Does smoking cause lung cancer? It seems likely that increased consumption of sugar during the last 100 years has had something to do with the great increase of these diseases during that time. Just because the exact sequence of causes and effects cannot always be determined is no reason to deny the probability. Eat lots of sugar if you like, but no one can help you lose weight and keep it off if you do.

The other major processed food is white flour. Like sugar, it has been available to common folk for only about a hundred years, and it consists pretty much of pure starch. Processors take out the germ and take off the skin so you don't get the vitamins, minerals, and roughage. Of course, white bread is fortified. But the point I'm leading up to is that even if you avoided sugar but continued to eat processed white flour — something almost impossible to do unless you eat flour from a bag with a spoon — you would still be laying on a lot of fat quickly because starch turns into sugar in the digestive process. Like sugar, white flour is almost void of any nutritional element other than calories, *lots* of bare calories easily assimilated into your fat system.

Knock off all processed sugar and processed flour. This means spurning almost all processed foods because, as I say, almost all of them contain either sugar or white flour. Eat whole-grain breads. But be sure to read the labels. You will learn that even "whole-wheat" bread sometimes contains white flour. Of course, whole-grain breads contain starch that turns to sugar, too, but at least they provide needed roughage at the same time. As for sugar, be advised that brown sugar, fruit sugar, turbino sugar, raw sugar, molasses, syrup, and honey are all sugar. Yes, I know honey is natural, but it is also processed. Bees process it: that is, they extract it from sweet flower nectar and refine it into honey. Give up honey. And grit your teeth, because for some of you, the worst is yet to come.

What do you put in your coffee or tea? Milk? Lemon? Alcohol? A bit of brandy in your coffee? Alas, alcohol is right in there with sugar and white flour, but I *am* trying to be reasonable, and since most American adults drink, all I can say is count the calories. I don't advise a diet of 900 calories of beer a day, but it has been done. It isn't good to drink beer alone. Wine is loaded with sugar. Well, it's up to you.

Instead of processed foods containing sugar and white flour, you eat fresh vegetables, raw or lightly cooked. Don't add sugar. Eat whole-grain breads and pastas, eggs, milk, cheese, fresh meat and fish.

What about butter, oil, and lard? Fatty meats? Your body needs fat, you know. Go ahead and eat them. Just count the calories. If you stay on your diet, whether to lose weight or to maintain it, you aren't likely to eat enough fat to hurt yourself. Some crank diets consist only of meat and fat, and of course Eskimos once were quite healthy on nothing else. We fixed the Eskimos by exporting sugar and white flour (and smallpox) to the Arctic Circle.

Eat meat. Deep-fry it if you will. Just count the calories. I don't ask you to be a vegetarian, but you will find that you can eat more food if you concentrate on vegetables and cut down on meat and fat. If you are used to eating a lot, you may find that high-bulk, low-calorie foods weigh heavily on the scale of desirability when you're on your diet.

The crucial thing, the radical thing, the thing that makes this hard enough to be interesting and thus workable, is cutting out processed foods. You have to modify your behavior by eating less overall. But just cutting down on calories while eating the same old foods will not modify your eating behavior sufficiently to make you stay the course. Cutting out processed foods just might do it.

Now it is time to run back to your friends or the library or the bookstore to get more books, low-calorie cookbooks, natural-food cookbooks, no-sugar, no-white-flour cookbooks. Add these cookbooks to your library of inspirational literature. Read and think thin. You can lose weight and keep it off. People do. You will have to change most of your eating and cooking routines. Good. You're on your way to a wonderful world of new taste sensations.

I just heard my sister say, "Bull."

"Oreos and donuts and malted milks and Shakey's pizza," that's what she's saying.

OK, OK, I did not say it would be easy. At first it will be hell. *And that's what I'm counting on.* I mean, if you are not tough enough to go through the initial withdrawal symptoms, then buzz off. You don't get something for nothing. Most Americans can hardly conceive of going off processed foods. And sure, once you've been on your maintenance diet for several years, you can probably handle, say, a milkshake now and then. (It won't taste the same.) Right now it's cold turkey. Just knock off fat-full processed foods and go on from there. You want a new life, don't you? A wonderful new life at that sexy, perennial, steady, stable, new low weight? Well, then, do what I say.

It is not impossible. Of course, I know you go out

to dinner. Go, and eat what is set in front of you. You are not playing around this time, however, so please don't indulge in the dieter's game of one-upping the hostess as you refuse to eat the mashed potatoes and gravy, only to give in by taking a full serving of the chocolate pie. Try to eat less if you can without being conspicuous; refuse dessert if possible. If you blow it, you blow it. The real test is the next day.

Start over again. It will be painful. One helpful trick is to make sure before you go out that you leave only fresh fruit and vegetables in the refrigerator to snack on. If you don't keep powdered sugar donuts in the house, you can't pig out on them. You are always weakest after a feast, because you think that a bit more can't do much worse than has already been done. It can. A meal you have to eat to be civilized and social is one thing, but breaking your diet on your own can destroy all you have built up, like W. C. Fields's fatal glass of beer. So remove temptation.

You have children, so the house is full of junk food? They would be better off on your diet, too. Don't tell me, I know how hard it is, I tried. About the best advice I can give you is to make sure your spouse is on the diet, too. Then have only one child (two parents outnumber one child). Children raised on this diet will prefer it, at least for a while. When they get older, they will rebel. Fine, that's normal. You have to let them go sometime. Maybe later on they'll come back to the wisdom of your ways. If they've been on pro-cessed and junk foods for years before you started your

diet, remember that you were, too. You can try to
bring them around, but don't go to war with them
over it. They *will* grow up someday, and perhaps even
leave home (that's a family joke). In any event, nobody
can be forced to diet like this. You have to do it on
your own.

If you take someone out to dinner, try to pick a
natural-food or vegetarian or Chinese restaurant where
there is some chance of your keeping somewhere near
your diet. Did I say Chinese restaurant? White rice is
as bad as white flour. Watch out for couscous, too.

You will know that you are making progress when
you find that a raw carrot tastes very sweet. Peas have
a lot of natural sugar in them, have you noticed yet?
After a while you will tend toward salads (plain vinegar
and oil, please) simply because you need to stuff your
gut, and salads have a lot of bulk. Vegetables. Whole
grains. You are counting calories so carefully that you
begin to think twice before you blow a lot of them on
a small piece of meat. When you start finding that you
prefer vegetable casserole to a steak, you're on your
way. This fresh food routine forces your eating behavior away from the high-calorie meat, potatoes and
gravy, and pie most Americans grew up on. The vegetarian health books you are reading for inspiration
will tell you that cutting down on meat is healthy for
you. Probably it is, but that doesn't matter so much
by itself. What matters now is that you are making a
radical alteration in your eating habits. You have to,

if you are to maintain your desired weight once you get down to it. Have I already said that if you just cut down the quantity of what you have been eating before, you will eventually start eating just as much of the same old stuff again and gain back all the weight you have lost? I know I have said that. So I'll say it again. If you just cut down on what you have been eating before, you will eventually start eating just as much of the same old stuff again and gain back all the weight you have lost. That's the way inspirational writing goes, you know. Repetition, repetition, the same thing over and over again. And that is the way your old eating habits have been, isn't it? The same old foods over and over again. And what has been the result? Fat.

Fat! Fat! Fat!

Cut it out.

By now you may think that I'm a fanatic and want you to be one, too. Maybe. Maybe not. I *am* trying to turn you into a very committed person. If you are not absolutely determined to make this change, you won't make it. I am trying to help you. Put your mind to it. Do it. The rules are quite simple. Get off most processed foods, eat 900 calories a day until you reach your desired weight (when you are forced to break your diet or when you have a relapse, buckle down and start over again), and then increase calories until you reach your maintenance level, and stay there. The change to fresh foods will wean you off your old eating habits, and before long — a year or two — you will find that your new diet really does satisfy your reformed appetite.

Yes, it will take years. But it gives you something to do, doesn't it? And if it is worth doing, so what if it takes years? You knew it wasn't easy before you opened this book. In fact, you know that it may be one of the hardest things you've ever done in your life.

Now some philosophy. Don't you want to have done something difficult in your life? It may seem a rather small thing to be proud of, if you are a 5′3″ female, say, and have managed to stay at 110 pounds for five years, ten years, twenty years. Especially when there are women 5′3″ tall, weighing 110 pounds, who never thought about what they ate in their lives. What counts is that it's hard for you. If you can't take satisfaction in knowing how hard it is to do something difficult, and in having *done* it, then forget it.

I'm not begging you to do this. I'm just writing the first chapter of a book on life and what it all means, and it turns out that what clutters the unexamined life is, you guessed it: fat. Everybody in America relates to fat these days. The worry about being overweight is largely a pseudo-fret, as I have shown, but there is something under it. *Somebody* out there is putting a lot of pressure on us to lose weight. If this diet appeals to you, try it. Whether you do or not, keep reading about it. It's inspirational. And it has a certain form we can use.

If you succeed, you will be entirely different from the usual American dieter. The norm is up and down, up and down. These people have a lot of fun with their ostentatious periodic diets. Diet talk fills up space at American cocktail parties, and that's helpful. You can tell people all about your diet over white wine, skimmed-milk cheese, and wheat thins.

There is a qualitative difference between what I'm offering and the usual diet game. How likely do I think it is that many people will take me up on this challenge? Not very likely. Not many people. That doesn't matter. There will be a few. Like world-class marathon running, this is not the sort of thing that many people are going to go for. But it is worth doing, just for the doing of it. Is it you?

Before you answer, let's consider another question. What *does* fat mean in America today? Throughout history a fat baby has been a healthy baby. Fat men were rich, and fat women sexy. Gluttony is one of the seven deadly sins, but the Christian middle class in Europe and America has overwhelmingly outweighed any other class one-for-one ever since the industrial revolution. Walk through the shopping centers and restaurants of middle America today. The men have bellies like barrels, the women arms like hams. They eat, eat, and eat. Where can you see their like? Women in Greece. Men in Germany. These are big people. Their backsides come one to a bushel, and not one in a hundred of them has read a book on losing weight.

For the masses, for the proletariat, for the workers and bourgeoisie, fat means affluence. Fat people are made fun of on television, but the real hee-haws are for people on diets. It stands to reason: if you can afford it, you would be a fool not to eat good.

Who, then, are the millions who read diet books? Of what class? Movie stars? Jet setters? The rich, powerful, and visible? Some, but mostly the same middle classes, city folk. Still, dieters crosscut all income brackets and geographical boundaries. What's the matter with them?

They can't all be frightened by scare tactics used by those in the diet and health-food industries who profit from this obsession with fat. Look how many Americans have successfully stopped smoking. These are people running scared. Now consider how many people manage to change their lives in a similarly drastic fashion by losing weight and keeping it off. Very few. Is maintaining a diet any more of a change of life than stopping smoking, any more difficult? You wouldn't think so, but count your friends. A lot more of them have successfully quit smoking than have kept off weight. I don't think many of them take their dieting seriously. They are not running scared.

Fat does have a bad press, though. Some even say that fat equals death. They exaggerate. Of course, extra weight does strain the system. Your muscles and organs have to work harder when there is all that fat to maintain and carry around. A strain on the heart, they say. And there are those plaques of cholesterol, packing up your blood vessels, breaking loose and clogging the bloodstream. Cholesterol has a mixed press these days. What seems to be settling out is what we knew all along: the body has to have fat, and if you don't eat cholesterol, you will manufacture it internally. People with high cholesterol counts do have heart attacks. There is a causal relation here more easily traceable than the track from that first cigarette to death from lung cancer. But you don't have to smoke. You've got to eat.

In the past, East and West, fat always meant life, fertility, beauty, health, happiness, and joy. Today you hear people saying such things as: "A fat ugly man." "She lay there like a mound of fat." "There goes old lard-ass." Yes, these do ring true. *They* have put across the notion that fat is ugly, which leads to the pop-psychology notion that a lot of fat is defensive. It protects shy boys and girls from having to interact as sexual beings with other girls and boys. Wives put on fat to turn off their husbands, who read *Playboy* (but did you ever see a skinny Bunny?). Men get fat so they won't have to fulfill their marital duties. How about fat as a sexual turnoff? It sounds good, but I doubt that it cuts the birthrate. The fact is that in times of famine, women quit ovulating. What is truly ugly and the true sign of death is emaciation.

I think this is why people often don't take fat very seriously as a threat. They recognize it as a sign of well-being. As people mature and get on in life, they just naturally get bigger. Nervous, skinny people are annoying. Even if they advance in the world, they don't seem quite to have made it. My brother (a China scholar) would ask: "What's wrong with them? If they're so rich and successful, why aren't they fat?"

Yes, the good things about fat seem to be too strong for most people to resist. To resist? Isn't there something wrong in a culture where the traditional image of the good life is denied? Anybody who has to ask what it all means is in trouble. And a culture in which millions of people are alienated from fat is also in trouble.

We'll come back to this. Meanwhile, back at the fat farm . . .

When someone trains for the marathon, he or she does not pay much attention to pop psychology like the above. I'll talk about running in a later chapter, but now I want simply to remark that readers who have seriously decided to fight fat have probably yawned their way through the last few paragraphs. It does not matter what fat means or has always meant, nor that one is healthier in the lower weight range than in the upper, all else being equal (which it never is, but no matter). It just does not concern the serious weight watcher that the rest of the world can get along as slobs, any more than it matters to the marathon runner that the rest of the world walks or rides.

I approve of attacking fat because it is *there*. This battle harms no one. You who are fighting fat, take notice, be aware. A few of us out here appreciate what you are doing. We know how hard it is. They say 95 percent of the people who lose weight gain it back, and 90 percent gain back more than they lost. If you're really worried about fat, taking it off may lead to putting more on. With those statistics, success in keeping it off has world-class potential.

Carry on.

2
Food

PHILOSOPHERS sit and think a lot. I sat a long time in front of the typewriter trying to think if there is anything in the world that can give more lasting pleasure than good food. I think the answer is no. Descartes votes for friendship and conversation, but he always enjoyed them over a good meal. Freud says that our very dream of paradise stems from the enjoyment of sexual pleasure, and I would not deny it. Sex merits a chapter. But friendship and sexual pleasure would not last long if you didn't eat. You may think I'm making a logical blunder here. "Is not food," one of my colleagues asks, "merely fuel?" Being well nourished is a necessary condition for enjoying the pleasures of friendship and sex, but it is not a sufficient condition. Am I not confusing the dance floor with the dance?

No. This is one place (there are others) where logical analysis leads to a silly conclusion. Without good food, friendship languishes, and sex goes stale. Show me a person who does not think that good food is both the *sine qua non* and the well-marbled muscle of the good life, and I'll show you someone who thinks Velveeta is cheese.

Yes, I know you want to know how long you have to stay on that 900-calorie diet to reach your desired weight. Let a philosopher tell you that it will take longer than any of the other books say.

Most readers of this book are obsessed with food. Nobody who toys with the notion of taking off weight can think of anything else. More cookbooks are sold than bibles. Yet there are people like my colleague who think food is just fuel and who walk down the street and pick restaurants with such remarks as, "That place looks cheap, let's go there." Most Americans don't know any better. The heart of one of Henry Miller's best books, *Remember to Remember*, is an attack on white bread. For him white bread symbolizes America, a place so uncivilized that people would put something with the consistency of cotton and the taste of cardboard into their mouths, masticate it into a dough ball, and swallow it. How can civilized human beings eat Wonder Bread? You and I were raised on it. We spread margarine and artificial grape jelly on it and smeared our faces. We didn't know any better.

Before I tell you when you can go off your 900-calorie diet, I have to distinguish good food from bad. Your ordinary fat person does not eat good food. Oh, the fatties start with good ingredients: potatoes, chicken, apples, fresh vegetables. But if you chop up the potatoes and vegetables and fry them; smear a paste of dough on pieces of chicken and fry them; cut up the apples into a paste made of water, sugar, and cornstarch and bake that glop in a shell made of white flour and Crisco; salt the chicken and french fries heavily and dip them in tomato jam; put on your apple pie a big dip of ice cream made from air, sugar, vegetable oils, and stabilizers that never saw the inside of a cow — if you eat all that, then you have destroyed your appetite. And your palate.

Nobody denies that you like this food. You can eat other things, but you prefer meat and potatoes. In my childhood in Iowa, shrimp was a smelly mess the local butcher sold for catfish bait. Then french-fried shrimp swept the country. Now you can get chicken, ham, or shrimp in every small town in America. Even my mother will eat shrimp if she has to. Besides shrimp, I can remember the first time I ever tasted pizza. I gagged. So did my sister and brother. We learned to eat pizza. My mother still won't touch it, can't stand the smell.

Innovations in food can be survived. You can even learn to like most vegetables. Food habits are indeed strong, but they can be changed. Shrimp and pizza were pretty wild for country kids raised on ham, chicken, and minute steak, but we got our arms around them.

Just how was the move made from fried chicken to fried shrimp and pizza? Through salt and sugar. French-fried shrimp taste much the same as french-fried potatoes if you forget the smell and dip them in sweet ketchup. People eat french fries for the salt, anyway, and if they eat something salty enough, they can even drink American beer. As for the pizza, the dough base reminds you of apple pie. (The first time I ever heard of pizza was when Dean Martin sang about his mamma's pizza pie in a movie with Jerry Lewis. I assumed that it *was* pie.) Pizza is salt pie. Where I live some of it is also sweet because they mix sugar with the tomato sauce and the pastry shell. Even so, Americans were not easily converted to shrimp and pizza. Most still prefer hamburgers and french fries, with ketchup, of course.

Human beings will eat anything if you just put enough salt or sugar or both on it. Salt and sugar stimulate your appetite while destroying your taste for anything but salt and sugar.

When you cut out processed foods, don't use sugar, and go easy on the salt, all that fresh food tastes flat and bland at first. You will learn to eat and crave it, but it won't be as easy as learning to eat french-fried shrimp and pizza. Soon, however, your taste buds will recover from the heavy salt and sugar insult, and you will begin to taste other things. Some people never experience the variety of tastes in the foods of this world. The philosopher's diet opens a new world of taste.

It's punishing at first? Did Maurice Herzog complain about losing a few fingers and toes in becoming the first to climb Annapurna? He did not. Don't complain.

This time, let's consider an adult male 5′8″ tall who weighs 170 pounds and wants to weigh 145. I put the 5′3″ woman on a 900-calorie diet, but a 5′8″ male can start with a 1200-calorie diet. Assuming that his maintenance diet is between 2000 and 2400 calories a day, how long will it take him to lose 25 pounds? Fat weighs in at 3500 calories a pound. Thus, with water-balance adjustments and exercise and metabolic variations, on 1200 calories a day, our subject can probably lose a solid pound about every three days. At that rate, allow for two and a half months, seventy-five days, to lose 25 pounds.

Don't you believe it for a minute. You have to go to dinner with friends. If you don't have a drink when you go on a business lunch, your client may think you are some kind of kook. You honestly forget and have your usual coffee and sweet roll when the wagon comes around. Monday night: football, beer.

What to do? Bear with it. Keep track of the calories, and when you go over one day, cut down to less than 1200 calories the next day. It won't hurt you — if you are a normal, healthy adult — to go one or even two or three days without any food at all. Fasting makes you feel weak and gives you a headache? It sure does. I don't recommend it. But it is an interesting experience for someone who is obsessed with food and has always had enough to eat. Dick Gregory says that after a week or so you lose all your appetite, and then it is easy to continue the fast. Perhaps. But unless you are on a hunger strike for a very good cause, forget fasting for more than a day at a time.

Let's eat; after all, that's what God put us here for, isn't it? Try to stay off processed foods, and try to stay on 1200 calories a day. Unless you go into hibernation, it is not going to take two and a half months to lose 25 pounds. It may take a year. Slow loss is better for you, anyway. Only if you are impatient enough to crash it can you do it in two and a half months. If you do crash, it will then be harder to keep your weight down than if you took a year to get there, because crashers bounce.

If you keep at it, eventually, *eventually*, you will begin to be able to handle the diet. It is hard to turn down desserts, but people do and you can. The worst thing may be that nobody particularly notices your heroism. You can also learn to nurse a drink.

Why learn to nurse a drink? Actually, I now am fairly certain that it is not true that alcohol, as my Grandma Penwell taught me, is the surest sign of Satan on this earth. Like sugar, however, alcohol is full of shamelessly naked calories. Sugar, white flour, and alcohol are so refined that they either fill your energy needs by burning up quickly so your body converts the other food you eat into fat, or they themselves convert at once to fat. It takes your body longer to embrace decent calories dressed up in fruit and vegetables, but if you eat enough of them, they will go to fat, too.

Now you begin to establish a routine of eating some foods and not others. At first you may feel uneasy about having a salad at a business lunch. Don't worry: nobody notices today. Oh, some people may still make tired remarks about rabbit food, but we've come a long way in this country. People are more tolerant about what other people eat than they used to be. Of course, if you want to cut down your appetite by smoking, you may have to go to the rest room to do it.

Even after you have established the salad routine, you have to expect setbacks. There may come a time when you say the hell with it and go back to your old ways for a month. It would be, in fact, a lot easier for you to maintain this diet if you could live in a monastery cell where exactly 1200 calories — no more, no less — were provided each day for seventy-five days. It would be easier because the monastery would impose a nearly total change in your way of life. Suppose you did it. Once you got back to the office you wouldn't last a day. Slow changes in your ordinary world are best. Determine in the depths of your being that no matter the setbacks or relapses, you will reach your weight goal and stay there.

This is an existential choice, by the way. Sartre says that each of us is responsible for what he or she is. If you are some kind of pervert, it is self-deceptive to blame it on your parents or society. You choose your own self. Sartre may go a little far in saying that a man with a clubfoot is to blame for being clubfooted, that he wants it that way. What about being fat? Did you choose to be fat?

Spinoza states the extreme opposite of the existentialist's total freedom and responsibility. Spinoza says that everything you do is absolutely determined, and that freedom consists in assenting to what you must do — and then you're responsible for being what you couldn't avoid being. That's called double-think.

Descartes, as usual, counsels prudent realism. The father of modern philosophy says that you should change your opinions and desires to fit the world only when you cannot change the world to fit your desires and opinions. It would appear that you can lose 20 pounds and then maintain the weight you reach, by responsible, free choice.

Can't you?

You understand that I'm taking you away from your mamma. Actually, I don't really care whether or not you leave home, but my little pretense here is that you have asked me how to take off a bit of fat and keep it off, and I'm taking you quite seriously. Your mamma taught you how to eat. She made you eat. Of course, you branched out later on. Maybe your mamma didn't teach you to drink beer. Your friends showed you a few things your mamma didn't tell you. And who taught your mamma? The advertising industry?

Processed foods are very convenient. I remember when TV dinners first came in. People would have them as a treat, like going to a restaurant (which in

Iowa is not such a dumb comparison). The world had begun to change. My mother used to win first prize for her angel food cake at the Taylor County Fair. My sister uses cake mixes. (These days my mother buys baked goods at the supermarket.) Get yourself a microwave oven, buy frozen and packaged foods, and you will never have to spend more than ten minutes preparing a meal again. This is a revolution. It gives you a lot of free time? I suppose it also helps absolve your mother of blame for your eating habits. Who is your mother to resist General Mills, Sara Lee, and the Jolly Green Giant?

What shall we do with that free time? If you are obsessed with food, the first thing you can do is pitch your microwave oven into the garbage and swear off processed foods. Second, zero in on cookbooks again.

I like ethnic regional cooking, myself. Provençal French, Northern Italian, Szechuan . . . Some of the vegetarian cookbooks are great. I recommend Mollie Katzen's *Moosewood Cookbook*. Take a lot of time picking out cookbooks. Read the prefaces, check out the recipes, look at the pictures. A lot of time.

You know the trick, don't you? You are spending hours obsessed with food without eating a bite. Think how much time you can spend with your obsession when you take three days preparing a cassoulet. Moreover, every dollar spent on cookbooks is a dollar that does not go for jelly beans. I know it's a tough choice in these tight times (the only taste I share unequivocally with Ronald Reagan is for jelly beans; hold the ketchup, please), but if you buy three cookbooks, you are going to think twice about the cost of one pound of jelly beans.

Obviously, begging, buying, or borrowing cookbooks is only the beginning. Can you cook these exotic foods in your old kitchen? Let's do what you've always wanted to do, remodel the kitchen. I'll just free-associate here and you can adapt the dream to your particular passions and situation.

If your kitchen is too small, it may be because of Frank Lloyd Wright. He was a great architect, but he designed kitchens like the galleys in small boats; no window, everything within arm's reach, and the joy of cooking be damned. I wonder if Frank Lloyd Wright didn't hate women, cooking, and perhaps even food. Look at a picture of him. He does look like one of those naturally skinny, dissatisfied people. Can anyone be happy who doesn't have a tendency to put on weight?

I'd have to knock out a wall and combine two rooms to get the size kitchen I want. This is so I can install a fireplace at one end of the room, something I'm eager to get to, but let's start with the floor. Brick? Or wide oak boards? Let's use boards for most of the floor, and put a lot of bricks around the fireplace. I'm torn about the fireplace. My predilection is for a huge square one with benches inside on either side, lots of frames and tongs for holding pots over the fire, and a rotisserie large enough to roast a wild boar. Too big, particularly for those of you who live in an apartment. We're not going to cook in the fireplace, anyway, so let's just make sure that it looks good and throws out a nice warmth on the tongue of brick that sticks out into the waxed boards. Is electric heat OK if you live in an apartment? Yes, so long as it throws out a nice glow. What you want is the glow.

A few chairs around the fireplace, and room for a small dining table in front of it.

Next, the stove. The place for the stove is against one of the side walls. How about a small restaurant stove, solid black, with four burners and a grill on top, two large ovens, and over it all a big copper hood with an exhaust fan? Fine. Out in the middle of the room, a couple of steps from the stove (room to move around in), set up a butcher-block worktable that you can walk all around. Above it, racks on which to hang pots and pans. The refrigerator and sink can go on the wall opposite the stove. Cabinets and counters along the side walls.

A word about the refrigerator: a normal-sized refrigerator with a standard freezer compartment is fine. You are not going to buy any frozen foods. You need the freezer for ice cubes.

How are we doing? We've spent (or contemplated spending) thousands of dollars on this project and have fussed around for months, obsessed with food, without cooking a thing.

You've not been cooking because you need an entire new set of cookware, the complete works. Not just ordinary pots and pans (although you need them, too), but woks and warmers and fish steamers and pâté molds.

Oyster openers, a set of graduated knives, a duck press, and a pasta machine.

Even Julia Child uses a Cuisinart these days, but I firmly advise you not to get one. First, there is the joy of chopping with a knife by hand, and second, chopping burns off calories. Every single one counts, you know. It would be pretty silly to have a big kitchen you can work up a sweat in, and then save work by having a Cuisinart. Besides that, a Cuisinart speeds up the preparation of food. The faster you prepare food, the sooner you have to eat it, and thus the less time you have to indulge your obsession without actually eating anything.

Have you been in a fancy kitchenware shop lately? Any one of them is good for hours. Before you buy, however, check out the local restaurant-supply house, where you bought (or mooned over) the neat restaurant stove. Such wonders for the kitchen, rugged, heavy-duty stuff that you can throw around to make a lot of noise and really occupy your kitchen when you cook!

There will come a day when your kitchen is ready. It may not have changed much if you can't afford remodeling (I can't). But at least we'll have it reorganized.

Many American men have cooked nothing more serious than fried baloney. Most American women learn to fry eggs. Now you learn to cook. My thesis in this book is that taking off 20 pounds and then maintaining the weight reached is a total change of life. Few people manage to do it because it requires a modification of behavior so radical and so interrelated with one's customs and habits, likes and dislikes, actions and passions, that few human beings can sustain it. You can't possibly just change your eating habits sufficiently to take off a few pounds and then maintain the new low weight. You must revolutionize your whole life plan.

Obviously it takes real conviction to do this, particularly since the American Medical Association assures us that being a few pounds overweight is not unhealthy, and because the concept of average weight is a pure abstraction from empirical data that may have nothing at all to do with health. Either you don't believe the American Medical Association and the United States Government, and think that you will be substantially healthier at the weight of *your* choice rather than at the weight of *their* choice, or you are reducing just for vanity's sake. If you are reducing merely to look better, you have to face the fact that even this requires a new way of life.

It is hard as hell to take it off and keep it off.

The way to contend with this need to change your life is to face the behavior problem straight on. Admit your obsession with food. If all you did before you began reading this book was eat a lot of food, you were not into food, you were merely stoking up. Now change from a glutton or gourmand, "a hearty or greedy eater," to a gourmet, "a connoisseur in eating." Furnish yourself with pleasant conditions for cooking, serving, and eating meals. Learn to cook difficult dishes from fresh ingredients. Subscribe to *Gourmet* magazine. Put bookcases in your kitchen for cookbooks and inspirational books like this one.

How am I doing? Yes, I know there are a few discrepancies to deal with. What is someone on 900 or 1200 calories a day doing dreaming about a kitchen outfitted to cook an ox? I'll get to that. What I mean is, how am I doing otherwise? If you don't eat up the kitchen plan, then you may not be truly obsessed with food. This obsession may be a prerequisite for every serious dieter. You see, the up-and-down dieters may forget about food periodically. They are not people obsessed with food, but with fat. Someone who is a periodic dieter, who screams, "Fat! Fat! Fat!," usually pronounced "Fet! Fet! Fet!" (an interesting combination of "fat" and "fed"), can't be helped with a dream kitchen and good food.

An obsession with food is a love affair. I'd much rather work with lovers of food than haters of fat. If you love food, you'll respond to kitchen dreams. But if you hate fat — something you can grab hold of and feel it being grabbed — then you hate yourself. And kitchens.

Is there any hope for the haters? Some, if they can be convinced that much of the talk and fret and bother about being fat is basically nonsense. If you are 20 pounds "overweight," the best thing might be to accept it and continue with your old ways. The problem, we all realize, is that you have been slowly gaining weight over the years, and you are afraid that 20 pounds now means 40 pounds five or ten years from now. You may

be right. I recommend the plan even if all you want
to do is maintain your present weight. The kitchen
hullabaloo provides at least a temporary diversion. Unless you change your eating habits *and* the food you
eat, you will continue to gain.

I can hear my sister clamoring to say that although
she knows perfectly well that I'm serious, this is really
one sweet time to recommend that anyone go out and
order a new kitchen. Look, I said I couldn't afford it
myself. But this is inspirational literature, remember?
Thomas à Kempis really didn't expect anyone to imitate Christ, either, nor did Immanuel Kant think anyone would give up telling lies, but they thought it
important to present ideals. So do I.

Consider the ideal. Most of us must keep our old
kitchens. Nevertheless, you can still change the way
you stock it and the way you use it. Cut out most
processed foods. Get new cookbooks. The basic goal
is the same. Change your behavior in the direction of
the ideal.

Even on 900 or 1200 calories a day you can eat good
food — not much until you establish your maintenance diet, but let's assume you've made it. More than
a year has gone by and you know your maintenance
diet. Suppose you're lucky: 2000 calories a day for the
5'3" woman and 2400 for the 5'8" man. You have a
lot still to learn about how to cook fine meals within
your caloric limits. More diversion.

Fine, but the crucial question now arises. Are you
stuck, like an ex-alcoholic, so that if you ever eat a

jelly bean or a powdered sugar donut you will soon
be right back where you were? No. For one thing,
you could never stick absolutely to your no-sugar, no-
white-flour, no-processed-foods diet without becoming as unpopular as a teetotaler in a bar. You have
learned to handle eating outside your kitchen and still
maintain your weight. You will still have binges and
breakdowns now and then, gain 10 pounds, despair.
But you know your life's project and you can do it.
After a week or a month you will go back down and
stay down.

The next step is learning to undertake controlled
deviations intentionally without depending on chance
and outside invitations to satisfy occasional needs to
eat something outrageously incompatible with your
maintenance diet. Exercise moderation.

How can anybody counsel moderation who, like me,
admits to a craving for jelly beans? Because if you do
manage to establish your new diet, you won't have to
choose; your body will thrust moderation upon you.

You have this craving to go down to the local pizza
joint and pig out on a giant special and a pitcher of
beer. All right. Do it. You will find it doesn't taste
the way you remember it. The pizza is too sweet and
too salty and there is too much of it. Go ahead and
eat more of it than you want. Go to bed with an
uncomfortable stomach. Cut down on your caloric intake the next day. By the time you go to bed the next
night, you will have decided grumpily that pigging out
wasn't worth it.

But damn it, you have to have a respite.

Right.

Before we get to it, let me tell you about my own experience. I read a lot, and when I do I can sit quietly eating cheap candy. I never liked chocolate much, but I love, loved — it's hard to tell these days, but let's just say that there are times when I crave — cheap candy. What I like are the obsessively mentioned jelly beans, none of those expensive substitutes from fancy candy stores, but the good, solid, old-fashioned kind from the dime stores of my youth. Yellow marshmallow peanuts, orange slices, red hots, and candy corn. Best of all: licorice allsorts. I once could finish a pound of cheap candy without noticing it, absently reaching around in the bag with disappointment when it was all gone. When the manufacturers slyly went up to pound-and-a-half bags, I didn't even notice. I remember quite well once eating the entire contents of a two-pound bag of orange slices in one sitting, but I forget what I was reading at the time. My wife prefers pigging out on potato chips, powdered sugar donuts, and Hydrox cookies, or even on Oreos if nothing else is available. She still never could eat as much junk as I could. Because my mother's cakes, cookies, and pies were so good, I never really liked store-bought pastries, but I could always finish a package if it happened to be lying around open and going to waste.

I say I can't figure out what my cravings are now, for although I go up and down, I've pursued the no-processed-food, no-sugar, et cetera, routine for long enough periods to alter my tastes. How you perceive food follows from your altered food-eating behavior. By altering your behavior you can even alter your beliefs.

It goes something like this. Pascal was a contemporary of Descartes's and both of them were mathematical geniuses. Descartes used his genius to apply mathematical methods to philosophy, but Pascal soon became convinced that there is an enormous break between reason (of which mathematics is the crowning glory) and faith (by which he meant belief in Christian dogma). Pascal's problem was that he was too smart. Christian dogma contains a number of flagrant contradictions, such as: that the same thing is both one and three things (the Trinity), that the same thing can be in many places at once at the same time (the Eucharist), and that something can be both human and divine (Christ). The logical Pascal began to doubt the Christian religion, and this *did* worry him, for doubt leads to disbelief, which would jeopardize the salvation of his soul. Pascal thus tried to convert himself to belief by setting up what has become known as Pascal's Wager.

Suppose the Christian God exists and you do not believe in Him. You've had it. On the other hand, if God does not exist and you do believe in Him, you've lost nothing. If God exists and you die a disbeliever, you will go to hell; but if there is no God and you die a believer, you won't know the difference. The smart gambler believes in God. You have everything to gain and nothing to lose, according to Pascal.

Losing 20 pounds and keeping them off won't save your soul, but it won't hurt you. The wager is that in the long run you'll look better, feel better, and be healthier. In the long run you're dead, of course, and then it won't matter how the gamble comes out. But would this be enough to make you a believer? No, and the wager wasn't adequate to make Pascal a believer, either. It is just not enough to will yourself to believe certain things, particularly contradictions. Pascal added further instructions.

Go to church every morning and go through all the motions of a believer. Do this without fail year in and year out, and lo, one morning you will wake up and find that you have faith. As a believer, when you sample a taste of disbelief again, you will find it repugnant.

With all due respect, I find that the same thing has happened to me with jelly beans, and, what is worse, licorice allsorts, which now taste like some sort of coal-tar concentrate. The cheap candy binges I've been on since my taste changed have been cruel disappointments. I choke the stuff down after the first three or four pieces, thinking I owe it to the person I once was. This candy is now too sweet. It also has a metallic or chemical taste. Those dyes, those artificial flavors — something has ruined the cheap candy of my childhood.

In his maturity, Pascal rejected and then periodically returned to the mathematics and logic of his youth in the same way. I now find fresh fruit vastly superior to cheap candy in taste and goodness, but was Pascal right to give up logic for faith? I don't think so, but it made him feel good. May he rest in peace.

Surely improving one's looks differs in life-concern magnitude from a desire to save one's soul. Pascal gained faith at the loss of reason, but need we go so far just to lose weight? Such extremism is not necessary. Let's consider what the great American pragmatist William James referred to as a moral holiday.

James said that in cases where there is no conclusive evidence either way, you can believe whichever of two alternatives you want to. Since no factual evidence can ever prove or disprove the existence of God, you can believe in God. That is taking a moral holiday. And you don't need to give up reason.

Again with all due respect, we, like James, are looking for a way to put our cake aside and eat it, too. We need not be extremists like Pascal, but the junk foods of our youth just won't do. They don't taste the way they used to, not if you've followed this diet. Go to any junk food outlet and try. I used to eat White Castle hamburgers. Unbelievable.

Instead of junk food binges, look for the best restaurant anywhere within a radius of a hundred miles. I grant you that this challenge may raise hoots of laughter if you live in rural Iowa. Today, however, most people live in large urban complexes, and wherever a million or more are gathered together in America, at least one decent restaurant can be found. If you can't find a good restaurant in your vicinity, join or start a gourmet club. Then once a month pig out on the best food within reach.

It may cost a pretty penny. You may have to drive two hours to get there (and two hours to get home). That's all right; it is time spent not eating food, but in the pursuit of it.

We dreamed a kitchen. Now dream a meal, the ideal meal. By clearing your palate of processed foods, you have opened the way to appreciation of an almost infinite variety of tastes. Like people who become connoisseurs of fine teas or wines, you can become a connoisseur of fine foods. As a gourmet, you can now go for the tastes. Go to France. To Lyon. The best chefs in the world cook in and near the city of Lyon.

Save your money. (This is cheaper than the kitchen. Once in a lifetime you might even do this one.) You and yours and another couple fly to Paris. Take the train to Lyon. Eat in a few good but inexpensive restaurants. Check around. Find out who and where the best chefs are. Consider their specialties and decide which one is likely to prepare a meal that would best suit you and your friends. Then go to the chef and press $1000 worth of francs into his hands. Tell him to prepare a meal to be served sometime during the next week. At his convenience. His choice of menu. You trust him implicitly. You place your palate in his hands.

And he will make you a believer.

It has been done. And $1000 for four is nothing. A

few years ago Craig Claiborne and a friend asked a chef in Paris to prepare for them "the finest dinner in Europe." The chef was Denis Lahana, who provided thirty-one dishes, nine wines, Calvados, and cognac. It cost $4000. (American Express paid for it as an advertising gimmick.) Let me hasten to say that I'll bet the food itself did not cost over $1000. Fine wine can cost a mint, and Claiborne likes wine. Most of us do not become connoisseurs of fine wines because we can't afford it, either the calories or the money. Tell your chef to go easy on the wine. It's his cooking you want.

If you can't afford France, try New Orleans.

3
Roughage

Let's get back to reality. Craig Claiborne was severely criticized for his excess. An episode of Fat Freddy's Cat drawn by the great underground comic-strip artist Robert Shelton condenses Claiborne's defense. Freddy's friend Harry chastises Freddy for keeping a cat. He says, "The average American spends enough each week on pet food to feed an entire family in Cambodia! Doesn't that make you feel ashamed of yourself?" Freddy thinks about it and then says, "No, because I'm sure a family of Cambodians wouldn't make near as good a pet!"

Some people accused Claiborne's critics of having no sense of humor. Claiborne asked rhetorically if anyone seriously believed that his dinner deprived anyone else of a square meal. The answer is that of course it did.

You, too, are going to be accused of frivolity, if not of immorality, because of your obsession with fat and food, so I want to prepare you to meet the challenge as best I can. Was it immoral of Craig Claiborne to eat that meal and cooperate with the executives who wrote off his expenses and used his little caper to advertise the use of American Express cards in exotic foreign travel? Yes. For private pleasure he expended money and resources that could have been contributed to the Cambodian Food Fund. On the other hand, that would not have encouraged traveling for pleasure, and tourist trade benefits the people of many countries. Which leaves us, with our French food fantasy, in what philosophers call a moral dilemma. The eighteenth-century philosopher Bernard Mandeville offered a way out. He argued that private vices lead to public benefits. A trickle-up theory of morality. It is awfully weak.

A few years ago I contributed a chapter to a book titled *World Hunger and Moral Obligation*. I put together the various figures about population, nutritional requirements, and food production around the world and concluded that if all the available food in the world were shared equally, then not just some of us but all of us would be undernourished. Numerous observers agree that this is still true today. Food distribution has to be unequal if some of us are to eat well.

Inequitable food distribution usually just causes undernourishment, but famines cause death. The threat of undernourishment and starvation throughout the ages is as good a reason as any why our obsessions about food are deep. The top priority of human existence — right along there with avoiding being eaten by bears and jaguars — is getting enough to eat today so you survive until tomorrow. Knowing that the exchange system that provides abundance for you results in others not getting enough, should you do something about it? Are you immoral if you don't? *Can* you do anything about it? It depends.

It depends in part on how serious you are about taking off weight and keeping it off. If you worry about my light tone turning into a sermon here, remember that this is inspirational reading, the hell and damnation part. After all, we might as well face the world we live in. Besides, I come to these interests naturally. Grandpa Watson was an itinerant evangelical minister of the gospel, and Grandpa Penwell was a farmer.

People of both the rich nations and the poor nations are obsessed with food. The way you tell them apart is that the rich are worried about eating too much and the poor too little. I concluded in *World Hunger and Moral Obligation* that we can produce enough food for everyone in the world to eat abundantly. All people in the world could be well nourished right now if everyone turned vegetarian and the grain crops were fed to humans rather than to beef cattle. I don't hold any particular brief for vegetarianism, although people on a no-processed-foods diet eat lots of fresh fruit, vegetables, and whole-grain bread, which reduces their desire for meat. Even in a well-fed world, people could eat some meat used sparingly, as in Chinese cooking. We don't eat everything on our plates, and a lot of pigs and chickens can be raised on garbage. And there are such animals as range-fed cattle, chickens, and sheep.

The problem is that nowhere in the world are business, government, and industry set up to distribute food equally. None of the world's leaders today could do it. It would take a world revolution to change the system.

Should you try to do something about it? Yes. This is a revolution I think we should all support. If anything is immoral, surely not trying to change a system of food production and distribution in which *you* are overfed while millions of others are starving is immoral. You can stop supporting the extravagances of the processed-food industries. You can eat less meat or even become a vegetarian. (I don't want to get off on this tangent, but commercial beef, pork, lamb, and poultry are so full of steroids, hormones, and antibiotics that even some meat producers say we should think twice about eating them.)

I have a colleague who used to say that his contribution to world civilization was in setting an example by living well. You can set an example by eating less meat and less food overall.

Don't expect instant results. You've got to learn to control your own fat before you can change the world. I am being quite serious. Roughage is a sobering topic.

Let's begin with water. Many people think that if they can just wring the water out of their cells, that will cut them down 10 or 15 pounds without losing any of the good stuff. Salt retains water, so they go off salt. This is all right. One needs a bit of salt, and there is no need to cut it out entirely in cooking — although if you do, you will get enough from vegetables. If you eat a lot of salt, it will be good for you to cut down, but it won't knock much weight off if you do.

Why not go to the source and simply cut down on water? People who do this end up with urinary infections. When on a diet, drink lots of water — as much as two quarts a day. Your body uses up fat, your kidneys filter out poisons, and you need plenty of water to flush out the kidneys. If you cut down drastically on water intake, the poisons will build up and you will get a kidney infection. So drink lots of water.

While you are at it, take a multiple-vitamin tablet every day; it won't hurt you. Do not take megavitamins, because large doses of some of them can poison you. Large doses of vitamin C are OK, by the way, because it is just ascorbic acid and is digested as a food. Why not take a 250-milligram tablet of vitamin C several times a day? It might even help prevent colds, taken with the right attitude.

As for vitamin C, a number of properly controlled scientific studies have shown that people who take massive doses of it — anywhere up to 15 grams a day — have a statistically significantly smaller number of colds than people who do not take massive doses of it. This evidence is as clear as the evidence that smoking causes cancer. You have to understand, however, that if people who take vitamin C have 1.0 percent fewer colds than those who do not take vitamin C, that is statistically significant. One study Linus Pauling cites shows that subjects who took 200 mg of vitamin C for six months had 13 percent fewer colds than a control group that did not. In some circles, 13 percent is a large number. As Pascal says, the results are desirable and you don't have anything to lose. No study has shown that eating a gram or two of ascorbic acid a day ever hurt anyone.

Do massive doses of vitamin C help prevent cancer? I don't know, but I must say that it gives me comfort to know that a fellow seeker of truth and health is a Nobel laureate. In philosophical terms, this is what is called a non sequitur. Just because Linus Pauling was very right once does not mean that he is right about vitamin C and cancer. Descartes warns you to check what the authorities say. On the other hand, Descartes was something of a fanatic about health himself. He recommended moderate eating and drinking, and he advised Princess Elizabeth of Bohemia on how to cure her constipation.

What the processed-food industry does to a grain of wheat is awesome. Basically, they take out everything that is good for you and leave an absolutely bland, easily digestible white powder that can be shaped into every possible form of pastry and packed as filler in almost any kind of food and library paste. This extraction gives rise to another entire industry of fortifying foods with vitamins and minerals that were there naturally but have been processed out.

They do not put back into white flour any of the

fiber that is essential as roughage for transporting wastes through your colon. Hamburgers and malted milks — most foods in the standard American diet — provide practically no roughage. Even a nice lettuce salad or two a day is woefully inadequate. One way to make up for this is to sprinkle a heaping tablespoon of bran onto some of your food during breakfast and dinner. Or you can drink it in a glass of water (straw tea; some people actually like it).

You eat cereal for breakfast? It is outrageous, but true, that not even the "bran" breakfast foods provide enough roughage. Worse, most of them are fortified with enormous amounts of sugar. You shouldn't eat those processed cereals, anyway. Just in case you think that All Bran breakfast food is all bran, get a box from the grocery shelf (for goodness sakes don't buy it) and read the list of ingredients. They appear with the item making up the largest percentage of the contents first, down to the item that makes up the smallest percentage. (Our quaint government regulations do not require processors to state the percentages; they just have to list them in order from highest to lowest.) Contents for a bottle of soda pop read: water, sugar, artificial flavor, artificial color, preservatives. Sugar stands high in all processed breakfast foods except Grape Nuts and Shredded Wheat, which contain no sugar. (Notice that Grape Nut Flakes contain a lot of sugar.) To continue the lesson, check a number of processed foods to see how manufacturers spread sugar content over several items. Sucrose, dextrose, corn syrup, raisin juice, and the like are sugar. Alas, as I've said before, honey is sugar. Honey is indeed a "natural food," but the substitution of honey for sugar does nothing but add flavor and raise the price.

There certainly are better ways to get enough roughage than by putting bran on your salad or drinking it in a glass of water. A philosopher's diet book should include at least one recipe: a recipe for bran muffins. If you make bran muffins from sugar-full All Bran with a recipe on the package that calls for even more sugar, you will not like my bran muffins at first. Try them. You will learn to love them.

The Philosopher's Recipe for Bran Muffins

Set the oven at 425 degrees. Grease a 6-hole muffin tin. Mix together dry:
   one cup of bran
   one-half cup of whole-wheat flour
   one-half cup of one of the following:
      whole-barley flour
      whole-rye flour
      whole-buckwheat flour
      whole-wheat flour
   one-half teaspoon of baking soda
   one-half teaspoon of baking powder
   a pinch of salt (optional)
Push the mix to one side of the bowl and into the space provided break
   one egg, add
   two tablespoons of animal or vegetable oil (e.g., butter, lard, safflower or corn oil).

Beat with a fork until egg yoke and white are mixed. Add
   one cup of yogurt or buttermilk or sour milk or sweet
   milk to the mix.
Stir with wooden spoon only enough to mix the ingredients
together once and so that everything is damp.
Spoon into muffin tin.
Bake from 20 to 24 minutes.

These muffins contain about 150 calories each. If you
eat two of them a day, you will get enough bran to fill
normal roughage requirements.

The way to make these muffins sweet, if you want, is
to add raisins or blueberries or any kind of dried or fresh
fruit. A mashed banana added to the mix makes the muffins
taste and smell delicious. You can add wheat flakes or oat
flakes or wheat germ or germinated whole grains or sun-
flower seeds or nuts. Better use an 8-hole tin if you add
much fruit.

I love bran muffins. Bran muffins constitute a world.
As you build it, however, remember to count the calories.

"Terrific, Doc," a dear deceased friend of mine would
have said. "You intend to change the world with bran
muffins."

Why not? Or if not the world, then at least the food-
processing and food-distribution industries.

Bran is the major form of roughage in the world.
Wherever whole-grain bread is a staple, statistically
relevant (a wonderful concept) evidence suggests not
only that bran helps prevent cancer of the stomach and
colon, but also almost every other intestinal ailment
known to humankind. Apparently it will not keep

women from getting pregnant nor improve the sperm count of men, but it will result in healthier babies.

Wastes must be fluffed up and eased through your colon by lots of moist roughage (drink lots of water), otherwise your stools become hard and keep poisons in your bowels overly long. You become constipated and have to strain to eliminate. The fiber people say that retention of poisons can lead to cancer, and that hard stools and straining can cause hemorrhoids. Even your doctor will agree that the irritation of bleeding hemorrhoids over the years can give rise to cancer. Your doctor may deny, however, that lack of fiber and lots of straining causes hemorrhoids. At the Washington University Medical School, I once asked a doctor whose specialty was operating on hemorrhoids what caused them. He laughed and said nobody knew.

People who live in parts of the world where a lot of roughage is eaten have fewer problems with hemorrhoids and rectal cancer than do Americans. Maybe they know something our doctors don't.

I do want to advise some caution about folk remedies. It is all very well to read a health book for inspiration, to keep one hopeful, and to supplement one's diet; but can all of those health-nut claims about seaweed and those wild accusations about the medical profession be true? Of course not. Doctors in general do not give you bad advice. Sometimes they don't advise certain programs because they know that most people won't follow them. Many of the programs they do offer are as good as any other. The trouble is, you have to follow the program to get results. One of Descartes's maxims is that when faced with the choice of various programs without much to go on to decide among them, you should choose one and stick to it rather than flit back and forth. Most American dieters flit.

Anyone with any brains at all understands that if sugar, white flour, and processed foods were in fact deadly, few people would now be alive. If vitamin C were a reliable preventive of colds, it would sell for ten times what you pay for it now. You know perfectly well that if massive doses of vitamin C or bran cut the incidence of cancer even by 13 percent, you could not buy anything edible in box, can, jar, or bottle not laced with vitamin C or bran. Members of the American Medical Association are not in conspiracy to destroy our health. Would that they were, for then you could easily figure out how to stay healthy. You could just do the opposite of what your doctor ordered.

Nevertheless, there is some truth in most health books, even the crankiest. (An exception that comes to mind is one about getting all the mucus out of your system. If you did, you'd be a mummy.) American medicine is curative, not preventive. In general, American doctors are trained to treat your symptoms, and many of them are much less likely to be able to tell you in detail how to remain healthy than are people trained in nutrition, health, and physical fitness. When you read health books, you have to filter out what seems reasonable.

It seems reasonable that the great modern increase in sugar consumption increases our susceptibility to some kinds of diseases. You don't need processed sugar, so it would seem to be a good bet to cut it out, although nobody knows for sure that sugar causes diabetes, arthritis, rheumatism, and neuralgia. Even doctors will tell you that excessive salt increases nervous tension and blood pressure, so it's reasonable to cut down on salt, whether or not you think salt causes menstrual cramps. As for the fiber connection, that is clear enough. Who wants to be constipated?

What about all the additives, artificial flavors, dyes, and preservatives in processed foods? As the Dow Chemical people say, everything is a chemical. And if you make a rat eat enough of anything, it's bound to get sick. Of course, some forms of cancer are caused by years and years of minor irritations by minor irritants (which is one reason causes of cancer are so hard to detect); and many additives put in processed foods to preserve them and make them look, feel, smell, and taste nice are minor irritants. Some natural components of foods are also minor irritants, but nothing in this world is perfect and nobody said you could avoid every possible cause of disease. Given the cumulative carcinogenic effect of minor irritants, and the fact that you can knock off a lot of them by avoiding processed foods, it does not seem unreasonable to do so, if you want to do as much as you can to preserve your health.

I digress. You won't complain if the philosopher's

diet introduces you to exotic new foods, tickles your palate, and improves your health. But the goal is permanent weight loss. Most people need inspiration and guidance to lose weight. Our conversation — I expect you to talk back — is meant to provide such help.

One reason for society's resistance to the revolution we are fomenting is that the change of behavior recommended here runs counter to almost everything that makes America tick. Consider who and what are very much opposed to cutting down on consumption. First, the processed-food industry and the advertising industry intertwined with it. Then agribusiness. Everyone knows that tomatoes, apples, oranges, and even many carrots sold in American supermarkets have practically no taste. To get good fruit and vegetables, you may start growing your own, or at least demand that different varieties be sold in supermarkets — varieties that need more care than the mass-produced items, and so must be nurtured by hand on small truck farms. This makes the big boys nervous.

Since the 1930s the trend in America has been to eliminate small farmers in favor of corporate agribusiness. My Grandpa Penwell was among the first to go under, so if you want to write me off as just another sorehead, go ahead. My grandfather loved farming. He wondered how I could think of doing anything else.

You know now what I mean when I say that your desire to take off a few pounds and keep them off makes you a flaming radical. The pressure you feel from society as a whole not to do it is very real. Your friends, everybody, all of America has a stake in your failure. This is a *consumer* society. A business society. The bottom line is not necessarily congruent with either your ideal weight or your health.

A French friend, green at the gills after he had driven across the U.S. eating in franchised restaurants all the way, once said to me, "Is there *nothing* that can be done to change the American diet?" Yes, Claude, I'm trying. But big business is right there waiting for me.

You know what happened to the hippies: they were commercialized. Hippie paraphernalia became a multi-million-dollar business. They thought they were a counterculture, but American society absorbed them. Today if you want to let it all hang out for a while, you can go to numerous commercialized encounter farms or workshops like Esalen, where you can pay plenty to play touch games, loll in hot tubs, stroll in the nude, even experiment with controlled substances and do other things you probably would not do back in Cedar Rapids.

Dieting is a profitable matter. Someone 5′5″ tall weighing 300 pounds had better see a doctor. But if you're only 20 or so pounds over the American average, then you are a setup. The scam is on, and not even people in the diet business want you to take it off and keep it off. If everybody did that, who would buy diet books and diet foods? Who would go to the fat farms?

It is a typical double bind. The diet industry draws

you in one direction, the food industries draw you in the other. The public helps the consumer industries. If you lose enough weight for it to be noticeable, more people tell you that you look awful than that you look good. Even the statistically significant number of those who say you look svelte rather than emaciated will be the first to notice when you gain it back.

I have two things going here. The lightweight banter follows from the basic truth that few people who fret about fat and diet are in trouble. Even if they exceed the American average by 20 or 30 pounds, the likelihood of their being struck down by some fat-caused disease is small. They suffer mostly from insults to their vanity. They see thin people on television, in movies, in magazine advertisements, and even in the flesh. The current American ideal of health, fitness, and beauty stands about 20 pounds under the American average. Thus a person who weighs 20 pounds over the average is 40 pounds "overweight." That makes much of the diet and health business a scam and an amusement: profitable to merchants, entertaining to customers, amusing to spectators. Many people view dieting the way they do murder and mayhem on television. They might not enjoy it so much if it were for real on their living-room floors. People pay plenty and get great enjoyment out of having the horrors over things they know won't hurt them. Being overweight in America is a lot of fun. Diet aids — low-calorie processed foods, diet workbooks, clothes for reducing in — are wonderful examples of what Thorstein Veblen called conspicuous consumption. How he would have exulted in the ability of American business to make a profit from people who are cutting down!

The heavyweight philosophizing has to do with taking control of your own life. There are many ways to do it. Since you are obsessed with food — which does not distinguish you much from the rest of the human race — we might as well start by seeing if you can gain control of your eating behavior. You want to take it off and keep it off. Fine. But if you can do that, the world had better watch out, because if you can succeed in this struggle, there are other difficult things you can do if you set your mind to it. Those other things may also go against the grain of government, business, and industry.

If you are serious about this, you are a troublemaker. Philosophers always make trouble. The powers-that-be dislike troublemakers.

Let's get on with it? OK.

How often should you weigh yourself? On the tenth, twentieth, and thirtieth of each month. You can amuse yourself on weight day, if you want. If you like to see the worst side of things, weigh yourself right after your largest meal of the day. If you like drama, don't eat at all the day before, and then weigh yourself just before your first meal on weight day. Mere play. It comes out the same in the end. Just be consistent and weigh yourself at the same time, under the same circumstances, every weight day.

When you reach your goal, start weighing yourself

once a day. Even if it has been impossible for you to keep to the set number of calories, if you have managed to get down to your goal, your diet contains fewer calories than are required for you to maintain your weight.

Remember I told you to count your calories? Now add up your records for the previous three or four months and divide by the number of days. If you are a 5′3″ woman and have been losing, your average daily intake probably was below 1600 or 1700 calories. Now increase 100 calories a week until you start to gain. The dividing point establishes your maintenance caloric intake.

Another way: when you reach your desired weight, if you are a woman, start eating 1800 calories a day; a man, 2000. That's 12,600 a week for a woman and 14,000 a week for a man. Divide it up any way you want. If you go out to dinner and eat 4500 calories at a sitting, then you must go back to your old 900- or 1200-calorie diet for a few days. That's OK. You've learned to juggle. Weigh yourself at the end of the week. Lucky you if you continue to lose. If you do, add 100 calories a week until you stabilize.

You remember that most women stabilize between 1800 and 2200, most men between 2000 and 2400. But there is nothing exact about those figures. Your maintenance diet depends in some part on how much exercise you get.

It is a scientific fact, alas, that as you grow older you shrink, and thus you need fewer calories to maintain your weight. And other factors count, such as the amount of sleep you get. You have to keep weighing and adjusting for the rest of your life. After many years, you won't need scales very often to tell where you stand.

I know that a number of you want to weigh yourselves every day from the beginning. Isn't that being a bit neurotic? Go ahead if you must, but the trouble is that your body tuning is not fine enough to be adjusted on a day-to-day basis. If you go to Shakey's for pizza and beer, and then to Baskin-Robbins for ice cream, you could step on the scales the next morning and find that you had gained 6 pounds. Does this mean, with fat at 3500 calories a pound, that you have to cut 21,000 calories out of your diet? No, that's ridiculous. Most of that 6 pounds will be lost through normal processes of elimination. Just cut your maintenance allowance in half until your weight is back down. The numbers are handy guides, but maintenance is never just a simple matter of finding a basic daily figure and then adding and subtracting. However long it took to get down to your desired weight, it will take much longer to get comfortable with your maintenance diet.

Do you know people who quit smoking years ago who admit that they still crave cigarettes? So do I. Will you be like that with jelly beans? I am. But you and I can do something the ex-smoker does not dare do: go out and buy a package and have a binge. Just count the calories. You also know ex-smokers who now cannot tolerate the smell of tobacco, and who gag when they go into a smoke-filled room. You may react to jelly beans like that, too, if you stay off processed foods, sugar, and white flour.

It is unlikely that you will ever entirely lose your craving for some childhood horror ("Jes gimme an R.C. and a moon pah": Calvin Trillin, *American Fried*) or your ability to enjoy a night out on junk food — unless you turn into a crank who sticks to the diet come what may. I advise you to follow another of Descartes's maxims: for getting along with people and being left alone, try not to stick out in the crowd. If you have to choose between eating something or making a confounded nuisance of yourself, *eat*. You will cheat some at first because you actually have to eat many fewer of the things offered than you might think. After a while people will consciously or unconsciously notice your food habits and meet them partway. When you find that people do not expect you to eat dessert (it's rather sad when that happens; you find you miss being asked to eat dessert almost as much as you miss eating it), you will know that by changing yourself you have begun to change the world.

Now can I talk about carrots? I have already remarked that after you have been off sugar for a while you will find that carrots are deliciously sweet. Carrots also provide a lot of roughage. You get the most vitamins if you just wash them, but the sweetness is enhanced if you scrape the skin off with a knife. Never peel a carrot. The best thing about carrots, however, is that raw ones take so long to eat. Serious dieters should begin dinner every night with two or three large raw carrots. Don't cut them up, bite pieces off. Chew each piece carefully. Diet books often tell you to take small bites, chew your food excessively, and even put your fork down between bites. The great thing about carrots is that if you do not chew them up carefully, you are likely to get a piece stuck in your windpipe — an unpleasant, even fatal experience. Carrots are not easy items to bolt down. So there you are, chewing away like a ruddy rabbit, and with as much pleasure. Carrots have a lot of bulk, a lot of water, and they are sweet. By the time you have eaten 100 calories of carrots — four *large* carrots or two chewed cups full — you have been eating a good long satisfying time and have diminished your appetite perceptibly. I won't bore you with how healthy they are. It would be hard not to say good things about carrots. Still, let me give the last word to the somber Austrian writer Peter Handke. "Don't eat carrots," he says in *The Weight of the World*, "they kill your desire for anything else."

You don't like carrots. Sigh. All right, all right. Try turnips. Cauliflower. Head lettuce. Raw potatoes, for that matter. Start your meal with raw vegetables that will keep you chewing and knock the edge off your appetite. Finish your meal with a banana. It is sweet, even cloying, and it ought to fill you up. Only 100 calories.

The raw-vegetable trick works even if you don't eat regular meals. There are mixed reports about whether you should. Some diets demand that you eat set meals at set times at set places, and never eat between meals. Even the thought of food outside mealtime is strictly forbidden. Such instructions are inhuman and impossible, like telling someone to think of sex only when doing it.

How about piecing through the day, 50 calories here, 50 calories there, every half an hour? The theory and the practice are great. You eat all the time, satisfy your oral cravings, and keep down sharp hunger pangs. Snacking may also very well be the way human beings ate for a couple of million years until they began to get civilized 5000 years ago and sat down for dinner. Be that as it may, piecemeal eating is pretty asocial today. I personally prefer to sit down to a nice meal and conversation with friends. True, I advocate a program that radically separates you from most people in our culture. If you do become a piecemealer, you will still have to eat regular meals often enough that you would be piling on more calories than your maintenance allowance. Nevertheless, the idea attracts me and makes a lot of sense, and I hate to let it go. Unless you want to opt out entirely, however, you had better stick to regular meal times.

And be happy that you can. Am I serious when I say you can set an example by eating less? Of course. We have to start somewhere, if only symbolically, if only as a gesture, to show that the overfed peoples of the world can get along on less. A symbolic gesture.

Oh, the beautiful complexity of that act! Let a philosopher rhapsodize. Just what *are* you doing when you follow the philosopher's diet? You are *at least* engaging in these human actions: cutting down on your consumption, changing your food habits, losing weight, improving your health, disrupting the processed-food industries, setting an example, refining your will-power, acting morally, fomenting a revolution, and changing the world. And that only begins to cover the complexity of your action. You may also be one-upping your best friend, rebelling against your parents, and — lest we forget — feeding your ego. Is there anything so wonderfully complex as a human action? Only the human mind itself.

You hear a lot these days about individuals not having much control of their lives. Corporate power is too strong, and we are helpless in our dependence on centralized production and distribution. Very well then, if you eliminate processed foods from your diet, you will have liberated yourself from forces that exercise immense control over the eating habits of the people of the entire Western world.

If you can develop the will to change and control your own eating habits apart from the norm imposed by society, you can think and act on your own as an individual in other matters as well. I don't see the problem of taking off a few pounds and keeping them off as trivial, not at all. I would like to think that John Locke, Jeremy Bentham, John Stuart Mill, and other great philosophers of individualism would agree with me. They wanted people to take control of their own lives. They urged people to persist, comprehend, and overcome. You may decide to go along with family, church, society, and state eventually, but you won't be free unless you have the personal power to take them or leave them. The experience of learning how to take off 20 pounds and keep them off is as good a way to begin as any.

One of the best things about this program is that it is like so much else in philosophy. It looks easy, its maxims are commonplace, it reiterates much that you already know. Yet, when you think about it — when you try to do it — it is harder than hell.

Don't be embarrassed at the seeming unimportance of your goal. What is important at this point is not your diet, but your commitment to it. People can't know what a project of exerting willpower is like or what it leads to until they commit themselves. At this point it is not the content of your act that counts, but that it is a difficult and long-term project freely chosen; not the seeming silliness of working so hard on such an ultimately minor matter, but how damnably hard it is to do, and that you manage to do it; not the content, but the form of the thing. For if you can do this, you can complete other difficult projects, the content of which may be far from minor.

So hang in there. And if you are not inspired by these last few paragraphs, you never will be.

OK, coach. Let's get on to running.

4
Running

Walk, jog, or run: it takes off about 75 calories a mile. If you move along steadily for four miles, you can use up 300 calories in thirty minutes or an hour, but that won't burn up a hamburger and a malted milk. The amount of weight you can lose through exercise is grossly exaggerated.

In fact, I finally sat down to write this book because a friend lent me a book in which the author claims that you can change your life with twelve to twenty minutes of exercise four days a week. That was the last straw.

Let me hasten to add that the book was *not* Kenneth Cooper's *Aerobics*, the greatest and most honest exercise book of all time. The author of the book that ticked me off does not even mention Cooper, although the only thing of any substance in his book is an abbreviated version of Cooper's program. (I even the score by not telling you the name of the offending book.) The purpose of Cooper's program is not to lose weight but to improve fitness. He advises you to undertake some continuous activity that gets your heartbeat up to something over 125 beats a minute for at least twenty minutes, or better, for thirty or thirty-five minutes a day. Cooper experimented on hundreds of thousands of U.S. Air Force personnel, and his conclusion — that sticking to the aerobics program cuts down your chances of having a heart attack — is supported by overwhelming statistics.

About the only activities strenuous enough to keep your heartbeat up continuously are running, swimming, bicycling, and rowing. Tennis and racquetball won't do it because your heartbeat drops during the pauses. You can't even keep it up long enough during a fast basketball game. As for playing baseball or softball, you might as well be lying down. Running and swimming are best, for about the only place you can be assured you are not going to have to slow down while riding a bicycle or rowing is in your own bedroom, on a stationary bike or rowing machine. And that is a real bore. Swimming does most for you because it stretches you out and exercises more muscles, but I find it boring to swim back and forth, and it does require a swimming pool in most climates. Running is the exercise of choice because you can do it anywhere (even around the deck of a ship) and it is the easiest way to get your heartbeat up and keep it there.

Read Cooper's book.

Cooper says you do not have to exercise every day to strengthen your heart, but what I read between his lines is that you should get your heartbeat up for at least thirty minutes a day, seven days a week. After every night's rest. If you miss a day now and then, no matter; but remember, this is for fitness — for weight loss, if you exercise only twelve to twenty minutes a day four times a week, which is Cooper's minimum, you might as well play golf.

Why do well-known doctors and athletes, and even Cooper himself, write blurbs for the dozens of books that give weak-kneed versions of the aerobics plan? The answer is twofold. First, all these people know perfectly well, as do you and I, that most Americans are not going to exercise much anyway. A book with a sensibly tough program — like this one — may turn people off. The books with weak programs are approved on the theory that some exercise is better than none, and every little bit of encouragement helps.

I don't entirely disagree. Even light exercise helps one lose *some* weight and keep it off. Seventy-five calories a mile does not sound like much, but when you are *shaving* calorie points, they add up. Suppose you run four miles a day at eight minutes a mile — a total of thirty-two minutes, which fits nicely into Cooper's aerobic program for heart and fitness. It also just qualifies you as a runner, for the dividing line between jogging and running is eight minutes a mile. And it uses up 300 calories. Do that for twelve days and the burnoff adds up to 3600 calories, a fair measure of a pound of fat. Do it for 240 days and you have lost twenty solid pounds.

Right?

Nah. You know that nothing in this weight game is that simple. For example, exercise supposedly reduces your appetite, and it does, if you try to eat right after running a marathon. But four miles at six, eight, or ten minutes a mile just tones you up, once you get used to it. You take a shower, bounce out singing, and are ready to eat everything on the table. You have to combat this urge.

The key point often brushed over or ignored in books that preach weight loss by exercise is this: you have to combine a decrease of caloric intake with the exercise. After you get through the agonies of establishing an exercise program, you are going to feel great, and when you feel great you are going to enjoy your food more. That may mean fat. Thus weight loss from regular exercise depends on your maintaining a set diet.

I did not want to say it at first, but the truth is that running four miles a day seven days a week is part of your program. If you run faster than eight minutes a mile, run farther than four miles until you have kept your heartbeat up something over thirty minutes. If you run slower than eight minutes a mile, plod on until you cover the four miles. Approximately thirty minutes on the road, ten minutes to get ready, twenty minutes to shower and dress. An hour a day. Seven days a week. Year after year.

Why?

If all you want to do is lose weight and keep it off,

not caring a hoot about your health and fitness, you just want to look good, then why this tedious physical-fitness routine?

To begin with, if it is vanity goading you, you *will* look better when you are physically fit. Your weight will readjust on your body as fat is replaced by muscle, your legs will take on a more defined shape, you could even stand straighter. You will also *feel* fit, and your fitness will be expressed in how you carry your body and by your beaming face.

That is not the reason that running is essential to your program. This program succeeds because it changes your life. Changing your dietary habits is not enough: you also need another project to take your mind off food, one which, keeping the goal in mind, helps you take weight off and keep it off. The routine of running — easier to establish than changing your food habits — does all that. You will get flak from some of your fat and sedentary friends, but there are so many people out there jogging these days that no one will notice you in the crowd. Some say running is a passing fad, but I think it is here to stay, like skiing. Human beings are, after all, large, heavily muscled animals. For millions of years our ancestors roamed the bush gathering wild fruit and vegetables and grains (a diet not too unlike the one I am prescribing) and running down other animals for food. Only about 10,000 years ago did we begin to domesticate animals and plants so we wouldn't have to chase them. Our muscles are the same and the instincts are still there, so it is not sur-

prising to find that millions of people enjoy getting out
to jog in the open. Running will survive. It satisfies
our primordial instincts. (Man the hunter? I run in a
local park on no set route, searching for cans and bottles, which I pounce on, pick up, and slam-dunk into
the nearest trash can. Spectators sometimes cheer.)

Running, satisfying as it may be, is not in itself
enough to dwell upon. Here the important thing is
form: one hour committed seven days a week to a
single, unitary activity. Compulsive? Listen, unless
you do something like this every day, year in and year
out, religiously, you don't know what compulsive is.
I don't want to get testy, but in teaching I find that
kids have watched television so much their attention
spans seldom exceed three minutes. Between com-
mercials. I have a friend in Washington who says nobody in government can be bothered with problems
that take more than fifteen minutes to comprehend and
solve. I would like to think that things are not quite
that bad, but such a short attention span might explain
some of the stupid things our leaders do. Short and
simple forms seldom fit the issues of real life. (Fill out
the short form, the 1040A, say, and you'll get cheated.)
We must learn persistence in contending with complex
detail. The form fit for shaping a life requires devotion
over the long run to the vision of a distant goal.

I want to focus your mind on a method of solving
long-term problems. Can you commit one hour a day,
seven days a week, for years on end? Try it by setting

out to run thirty minutes a day, no exceptions. See if you can.

You may well ask, OK, smart fellow, do you do it yourself? Yes. I do. Except when it is raining hard or is extremely cold, snowy, and icy or I have too much to do. And sometimes the tendon in my right leg . . .

If you can run five or six days a week at first, you'll be doing very well. The crucial thing is commitment. Taking your run is like turning down dessert. At first you eat dessert because you don't want to hurt your hostess's feelings. Later on you realize that she is perfectly happy if you don't eat dessert: she can feed it to her kids tomorrow. Anyone can find all kinds of reasons for not sparing an hour to run. There is only one way to stay on track: you must simply make running come first, *whatever* else there is to do. You must decide that nothing you do in a day is more important than taking an hour for your run.

What if you are the President of the United States and have very important things to do? Whoever you are, almost everything you do during the day may be — in substantive content — more important than running. Looking at the form of your day and your life puts a different light on this project. Suppose you want to write your memoirs (which, if you are President, you will). You have to arrange the time to do it.

We are working on the form of your life. I want you to learn to do one single, unitary thing at least one hour a day, day after day. Let's do it by returning to the content of the weight-loss program.

Most of us are awake at least sixteen hours a day. Reserve one of those hours for running.

Not only do you have to run, you have to keep track. Exercise makes a difference to your maintenance diet. If you run, you can raise your caloric intake a few points. Remember, however, if you miss a day of running, you use up 300 fewer calories that day and have to knock those calories off your diet. Again, the body is not tuned quite that finely, but in cumulative terms it all counts.

Add a few miles to catch up on those days you can run, although total mileage is not as important as the daily routine of taking an hour a day to run and count. It is an interesting exercise — I mean the problem of rearranging your life so you can spend an hour a day running. You could attempt this with any other single, unitary activity, an hour a day, seven days a week, but it happens that you want to lose some weight and keep it off. Running is part of the program. In the long run, you do it for the form of the thing, to learn how to take control of your life.

After a while you will find fewer and fewer excuses for not running every day. You won't miss more than a day or two a month. Once I went, as I recall, something over 200 days without missing a day. This beat the record of Joe Ullian, the running philosopher, providing a quiet philosopher's satisfaction for me and a somewhat louder philosopher's chagrin for Joe.

Don't overdo it trying to make up for lost days by increasing time and mileage on succeeding days. The point of the exercise is that it takes *only* an hour, just one hour, seven days a week. Instead of distorting your routine by taking much more than an hour, you can walk and use the stairs. Explore the world of stairways. All office buildings and hotels have them. Unless it is more than ten stories, you will usually beat the elevator. It is also unlikely that you cannot afford the time to walk anywhere you have to go within a mile. You can walk a mile at a fast clip in fifteen minutes, and easily in twenty minutes. If you live within two miles of your work, walk to and from work. Use the time to think about something. (I've thought about the distinguishing characteristic of philosophers, and I think it may be this: philosophers schedule time to think.)

But the run is still on! Even if you walk four miles round trip.

You may need help getting started, and in surviving the first six weeks of agony. First, get a thorough medical examination and a doctor's approval before you start running. If you are a normally healthy adult, there probably won't be any problem; but if you have not done much exercise since high school, you'll feel better (so will your spouse) if you have a stress test and get your heart checked before you begin. Doing all this also rules out a major excuse for not running: the worry that maybe you shouldn't.

Second, subscribe to *Runner's World*, or *The Runner*, or *Women's Sports*, or all of them, it doesn't matter which. They are absolutely full of inspirational literature every month.

Third, go to a sporting-goods store that has a large selection of running shoes and find a knowledgeable clerk. If you think the clerk is uninformed or trying to sell you a bill of goods, go to another store. Buy the shoes that feel the best. (They will be expensive.) This is important because you can hurt your feet and knees and back if you wear ill-fitting and inadequate shoes. Ordinary tennis shoes and sneakers are *not* adequate. They do not provide the support and cushion you need for your pounding heels.

Good running shoes are essential, but you don't need to buy another thing. You already have shorts, sweatshirts, T-shirts, and socks. You can run in jeans, slacks, or old corduroy pants just as easily as in the finest running suit money can buy. But that's my hang-up. If you want to run in Frank Shorter shorts and Joan Benoit shirts, buy. American track stars have to make a living, too.

Go slow. Do not exhaust yourself. If you get breathless, slow down. Walk until you recover. Pace yourself, because it is just as well to start out by covering the entire four miles. Oh yes, this is going to take more than an hour until you get up to eight minutes a mile. Beginning is the hardest month.

How you feel the next day depends on many things. If you have walked no farther than from the refrigerator to the television set for years, then you are going to feel very stiff and sore.

Very good. If it hurts, you're alive.

But . . .

If you can't make four miles the first day, don't destroy yourself over it. You have to begin where you have to begin. Let's hope you can do at least a mile. Record your distance and try again tomorrow.

You may be so stiff and sore on the second day that you can hardly walk. OK, do as much as you can. You will be able to feel how it goes. And the best thing for stiff and sore muscles is exercise and a hot bath or shower.

Your muscles are going to protest for at least three weeks. You will just have to carry on nevertheless.

If you smoke, you're in trouble. It would be best to quit, but I'm not going to bug you about that. I could tell you how to quit, but we can't do too much at once. Anyway, I've already told you how. It is a matter of different content (stopping smoking and staying off rather than losing weight and keeping it off) but same form (commitment).

About your wind: your lungs may burn at first. Slow down. Many people start out too fast. You are not going to be a sprinter, you are just working up to run a medium distance. You can't run four miles the way you run 100 yards. The name of this game is endurance, not speed. Just start slow and keep at it. If you get breathless, slow down. If your side aches, walk awhile. This will pass. In six or eight weeks you'll be breathing easily. Read Joe Henderson's classic *The Long Run Solution*. (Come to think of it, Joe Henderson — the premier writer and theoretician of the running revolution — was born in a small town in Iowa just a few miles north of my hometown. Could it be all that corn?)

Most people get over muscle soreness before they improve their wind, but after you have been running for a few years and then stop for a few months, when you start again your wind is usually fine but you have to go through the same sore-muscle routine all over again. Did I just come up with another reason to be faithful to your running routine? If you run every day, you won't have to endure the agony of getting your muscles back into shape when you start up again. Hmm.

Never mind. Once you begin, you are not going to miss more than a day or two at a time for years. As my sister-in-law, who was born in Illinois and schooled at the London School of Economics, says, in her best fake British accent, "You're going to stick to it, aren't you?" The "aren't you?" has a sarcastic lilt to it. Ignore that lilt. Nod and huff on. If you can talk while you are running (this defines aerobic running), then you reply, "I know I am, don't I?" Different words, but the lilt in the same place.

Did I say that the runner's world is another world? It is, and not one only of running. It is also a world of stretching — not high school and army calisthenics, but slow bends and holds. Many of the best exercises are based on yoga. You will have to fit some stretching exercises into your hour. Your hour already takes an hour and ten minutes? There is nothing sacred about sixty minutes. But if you stretch your hour into more than ninety minutes, you are doing more than the program requires. Experts differ on how long, but ten to fifteen minutes of stretching exercises before and after you run should keep you out of trouble.

The primary problem with running is that it strengthens and shortens some of the muscles in your legs and back differentially. You must stretch your muscles so that all of them are in balance. Otherwise, you may suffer muscle spasms in your back or strain the muscles in your legs in various ways. One of the best ways to stretch all the muscles is to swim. You could even swim every day rather than run. Running is less bother, and it is usually easier to find an open road than an open swimming pool.

I use four basic stretching exercises for legs and back:

1. Stand about three feet from a wall, lean over, and put your palms against the wall, keeping your legs straight and your feet flat on the floor. Hold three minutes. This stretches the backs of your legs.

2. Lie on your back, keep your legs straight, and hold your heels three inches off the floor for three minutes. This strengthens your stomach.

3. Lie on your back with your knees up and your arms crossed on your chest. Rise up as though doing a sit-up and hold three minutes at the point of greatest tension. This strengthens your stomach and back.

4. Stand with your legs straight, bend over, and touch

your toes (or try to). Hold three minutes. This stretches your legs and back.

Don't bounce. Don't do leg-ups or sit-ups or toe touches. Go to the positions of tension and hold. Slowly you will stretch out. Muscles in your legs, back, and stomach will stretch and strengthen into proper balance. There are many good exercises. Here is a chance for another orgy — on exercise books — at the library or bookstore.

If you run, you will have toe, arch, heel, ankle, shin, calf, knee, thigh, lower back, stomach, chest, neck, and head pains. Sometimes an excruciating pain will hit you in one place or another, and it is often a puzzle what to do about it. I once had an incredible pain in my ear — not inside, but in the flap. I did what most runners do, continued running, and it went away. Most of these pains disappear as mysteriously as they appear. Just carrying on seems to be best, if you can stand it. If it really is severe, you'll stop.

If a pain persists for several days, stop running for a while. A charley horse may take weeks to heal. If it gets very bad, see a doctor, who probably can't help much, but you will feel better knowing that. Make sure you go to a doctor who runs or who is sympathetic to running. You don't have to go to a doctor to be told that running is bad for you. Plenty of your friends have already told you that. What you want is a doctor like the one I saw once. (Runners love to hear and tell these stories.) I had an excruciating pain in my right knee. It felt as though there were a thumbtack under the kneecap, pointing in. I told an orthopedist (recommended by the university track coach) what my problem was.

"How much do you run?" he asked.

"Oh, five or six miles a day," I said.

"Uh-huh," he said, "let's x-ray it. Any other problems? How about your back: any lower back problems?"

I said that a few years ago I had come down hard on my right heel, which caused a severe lower back pain, but I got over it.

"Might as well x-ray that, too," he said. "You have medical insurance don't you?"

"Uh-huh," I replied.

"Your knee is OK," he said, as he stacked the X rays on a light frame, "but let me show you something about your back. See those vertebrae? Either you do run as much as you say or else you play for the Pittsburgh Steelers. A normal string of vertebrae line up evenly. But look at yours. Every one is jiggled out of line." He stood there tapping his teeth with a pencil while we looked at the X ray.

Finally I said, "Well, is that bad?"

"Oh," he replied, "probably not if it doesn't bother you. I found out what caused your lower back problem a few years ago," he went on. "See here," he pointed, "that little white line on the lower vertebra there. It's been cracked and healed. Didn't it hurt?"

"It hurt like hell," I said, "but I didn't have anything

that seemed like a pinched nerve, and I could move everything, so I didn't do anything about it."

"Doesn't matter," he said. "We couldn't have done anything about it anyway. You just let it heal, stay off it. I assume you did that?"

"I did," I said.

The doctor started wrapping things up.

"But look," I said, "what about it? Can I keep on running?"

"Sure, why not?" he asked.

"Well, my back, joints, all that wear and tear. Won't they wear out?"

He blurted out a laugh and said, "Not unless you intend to live to be a hundred and seventy-five."

"Tell me," I said as he started to go out the door, "do you run yourself?"

"Sure," he said.

My wife asked me if I really wanted to put that story in this book. "Those jiggled vertebrae give me the creeps," she said.

I include the story for a number of reasons. For one, I'm telling it like it is. If you run, you are going to have a number of problems. But you'll have different problems if you don't. It all balances out. I am quite convinced that keeping your heart and respiratory systems in great shape in exchange for sustaining some wear and tear on your joints is well worth it. Either way you are not going to live to be 175. Too bad: my father would have liked to.

In a well-managed running program, the chances of

hurting yourself badly are not as great as those of getting hurt in an automobile accident.

Now that I've given two fallacious arguments in a row, I'd better stop for a short philosophy lesson. Because you gain more heart repair by running than you lose in joint damage is no argument that you have to run. And because you do a dangerous thing like riding in automobiles is no argument that you should do a less dangerous thing like running. The conclusions in these implied arguments do not follow from the premises. They are non sequiturs. Health-nut literature is packed chock-full of such fallacies. You should reject them.

Cooper demonstrates in his *Aerobics* that the beneficial effect of running on your heart can be spectacular. This is no fallacy. But the common statement in running literature that nobody who ever finished a marathon has died of a heart attack is just not true (as James Fixx, who wrote *The Complete Book of Running*, spectacularly demonstrated); no more true than the nuclear industry's claim that nobody ever died of cancer caused by working in a nuclear power plant. Given the world we live in, your chances of dying from radiation are a lot greater than of conking off while running, *n'est-ce pas*? I say that you might as well stick to the program (even if the argument is a non sequitur).

Besides, as we all know, the point is to lose weight and keep it off. As long as the method does not hurt anyone else and does not hurt you all that much, what's the problem? You've got to do something with your life unless you want to just sit there (which is doing something, too, you understand). While the regimen I recommend for fulfillment of my program hurts, at least to begin with, it is unlikely to cause serious harm. In fact, if you have been inactive, you may be substantially healthier after you have followed this program than you were before, whether you want to be or not.

If you really do get into this program, you are probably going to want to tell people about it. Let me warn you that very few people care, and a remarkably large number of people actively do not want to know. Oh, you will find a few who are interested and willing to listen (tell them to buy the book), but even your seasoned jogger will probably begin to edge away if you expand on the virtues of going off processed foods. Remember again what Descartes said: it's best not to stir up the natives.

You are undertaking this program for yourself. If it leads to changing the world, fine, but you have to begin at home by changing yourself.

You will hear that some world-class marathon runners live on Twinkies and french fries, and drink lots of beer. I don't doubt that some of them do, although they may just be playing to the grandstand. Anyway, they don't run for their health.

No. Even when these guys are *not* running regularly they usually stay close to Van Aaken's ideal weight, which you recall is 20 percent off the American average. That means that a world-class marathoner 5′10″

tall is probably going to weigh 132 pounds or less. I've not said anything about body type because the perfectly healthy range of weights around the American average is something like 20 pounds in either direction, a range of 40 pounds. At the high end of that range, you will perhaps (but not necessarily) find the classic heavy, endomorphic body type; and at the low end, you will perhaps (but not necessarily) find the classic light, ectomorphic body type. Most people are in the middle, mesomorphic range, and a mesomorphic man 6′3″ tall could easily weigh either 180 or 220 pounds and be healthy. I don't want to make much of these figures because the ectomorph-mesomorph-endomorph body classification is not diagnostic. What I do want to point out is that many world-class marathoners have ectomorphic body types. (So does Christ in most representations of him, whereas Buddha is always a fat jolly endomorph, for whatever you want to make of that.)

If you run four miles and then want to blow the 300 calories you've burned by eating a Twinkie and drinking a can of beer, why not?

Not yet. Let's get the routine down first. Entrench your ability to stay off processed foods for a year or two before you start having periodic moral holidays. By then I'd hope that you'd decide to splurge on soufflé Grand Marnier rather than on Twinkies, and your beer would be dark, imported, and cost three times the price of a bottle of American light. I suppose that's basically an aesthetic prejudice on my part.

Besides the issue of body type, I have also been avoiding the question of whether or not some people naturally have metabolisms that burn up more calories than other people. There is indeed some variation, and why some people are fat and others thin may have more to do with their metabolisms than with their body types. When someone who is truly obese tells you that he or she is sticking to a 900-calorie diet and can't lose weight, however, you should follow the philosopher David Hume's counsel about reports of miracles. If only a few people give the report, you are to ask yourself which is more likely, that the miracle really occurred or that they are lying. If a vast multitude report a miracle, is it more likely that they were deceived than that the miracle occurred? I am sure there is no evidence whatever that fat people are more likely to lie than anyone else, but some fat people have been known to lie about how much food they eat. Probably as many thin people lie about how *much* they eat as fat people do about how *little*.

Thin people often appear to eat more than they do. If you know thin people who always seem to be snacking, it is probable that their daily caloric intake still does not exceed by much, if at all, the average maintenance diet for people of their height and weight. There certainly is some variation in the amount of calories different people burn to maintain given weights, but thin people who actually do eat like a horse eventually end up looking like one from behind.

David Hume did not deny the possibility that miracles may occur. He was just a suspicious fellow who would certainly understand our problem. In his youth he was gangling, thin, and earnest. Anyone would have classed him as an ectomorph. In his twenties he had a skeptical crisis, wrote one of the classics of Western philosophy (*A Treatise of Human Nature*), and gained 60 pounds in six weeks to become a fat, jolly fellow for the rest of his life. Hume was a wonderful man. He and Benjamin Franklin used to have grand times together in Paris, eating and drinking and playing whist, and pulling bluestocking ladies down to sit on their fat laps. Having looked like a classic ectomorph in his youth, and like a classic endomorph in his maturity, Hume would be the first to suggest that the likeliest cause for weight gain is not a sluggish metabolism but the total intake of food.

People do differ, but before you believe wild stories, get an honest calorie count. If you then find someone who weighs 100 pounds, eats 4000 calories a day, and cannot gain weight, or who weighs 300 pounds, eats 1000 calories a day, and cannot lose weight, then urge that person to see a doctor. You have discovered not a living miracle, but someone with an abnormal metabolic system who is very ill.

There is much more to say about running. If you like it, you will find it a wonderful thing. Some people say that running gives them a natural high, and if it does, this might explain why other people say running lifts them out of depression. In itself, running is something you can do for yourself for a lifetime. Whether or not you enter races, you can keep records of distances and times, set personal goals, and have a private world all your own of endeavor and accomplishment. All of that is fine, but it goes beyond the needs of our program. I leave the subject with some reluctance. Running, however, is something most people can tolerate but not everyone can like. If you simply cannot abide running, try swimming or bicycling or rowing instead (different content, same form). I now move on to something for which even the most sedentary of human beings is willing to raise a heartbeat. Only the rare human being does not enjoy sex.

But before going on, let me pause and look around. What a marvelous place the Center for Advanced Study in the Behavioral Sciences is for writing a book on how to take control of your life (self-imposed behavior modification, shall we call it?). The Center sits on a hill above Stanford University, from which one can look down across shining San Francisco Bay to the foggy Berkeley hills beyond. The philosopher George Berkeley wrote a poem that contains the line, "Westward the Course of Empire takes its Way," and that is why the town built up around the first great university on the West Coast was named Berkeley.

At dusk lights sparkle in a pattern of a million interlaced strings, over the hills west to the Pacific, across the salt flats north to San Francisco. The night is velvet and the dawn is pink and blue. In the sharp transparent light of midday, the miniature spires far away stand like one of Italo Calvino's magic cities seen through a hole in a gem-encrusted egg.

Just over the hill behind the Center is the Stanford Linear Accelerator. This building, a mile long, houses equipment for the study of the interior of the atom. It runs right beside the San Andreas Fault. In 1906 a slight movement along the San Andreas destroyed the city of San Francisco. It has happened many times in the past. It will happen again. Seismologists say that the earth will move under our feet before the end of the century. These are apocalyptic times. We wait for The Big One.

And the air tastes and sparkles like dry white wine. Every day is like early spring. My book is half done. Tomorrow is the Chinese New Year and I am going with friends to a Chinese banquet. We will talk and laugh and eat ourselves silly. We will ring in the Year of the Dog.

I look out the glass wall of my study across the rolling Stanford hills. When I arrived in September they were the smoothest of California golden tan. The squat black oaks were bare. Now it is late January of another year.

There has been rain. The oaks are green, the hills are green, brilliant emerald green, deep with richness and life. Towering ranges of cloud stand over the sensuous hills.

The hills beckon. I change into my running clothes, lace on my worn running shoes, step outside, and run.

5

Sex

SPEAKING of obsessions . . . like any normal human being, I've been obsessed with sex much of my life. It's an awfully difficult thing to get your hands on philosophically. Forgive me for making an attempt to do so in this book, a book about diet in the large sense, a book having to do with the form of life.

There are two major difficulties in approaching sex philosophically. One is to stay free of Freud, and the other is to avoid making — as my father used to say — a jackass of yourself. In another book I once wrote (*Sex and Revolution*, about which I'll say more later), my first chapter was titled "Plain and Fancy Fucking" — not about technique, the plain being for fun and the fancy involving love and hate. The epigraph for the book was "fuck" from Henry Miller's *Tropic of Cancer*, and I delved into the subject with great verve. That was in the mid-1960s, and more recently I tackled sex again in a novel about a love affair between a seventy-year-old man (preparing to set the world's record for over-seventy marathon runners — the record in running the marathon, that is) and a twenty-six-year-old woman.

There was some interest in the manuscript, so I found myself in a nice restaurant in New York City talking to a young woman in publishing. She was about thirty, she had read the manuscript, and she found *herself* sitting opposite this older man whose hair had obviously once been wild and red, but whose beard now is mostly white. She sat with her knees close together and told me that the novel was well written, but the age difference was absurd. Mid-life-crisis novels are big now, so I should change his age to forty, and then it might go.

"But the novel is about the ubiquity of love and the inevitability of death," I said. "The point is that their ages don't make any difference."

"But my *father* is seventy!" she said.

My eyes took on what I like to think of as a wicked gleam, but which comes across, I have been told, as a merry twinkle. "Oh?" I said. "And does your father turn around and look at women when they walk by?"

"Well, yes. He does," she said.

I sat back in my chair and held my hands out in a wonderful shrug of proven point. She went back to her office, and she told me later that an older woman there had said to her, "Listen, kid, I know some seventy-year-old men who are *all right*." Nevertheless, *Going the Distance* is (as my agent taught me to say) still "in progress."

Human beings are sexed, which does not distinguish them from other animals. But only humans are sexually arousable at times other than during the female's estrus period. Human beings, male and female, from puberty to the grave, are almost always interested in sex and need no special biological incentives to excite them. You knew that? All right, here is the question: what role does this unique and atypically general sexuality of human beings play in the complex working out of human destiny? Not just, What does it mean for the fate of humankind that we are sexed? but, What is the meaning of our being *over*sexed?

In philosophy it is not a cop-out to end with a question and not an answer. Here is a good definition of philosophy: getting the question right. For example: have I made a jackass of myself yet?

In *Civilization and Its Discontents*, Sigmund Freud says — and I believe him — that "sexual love has given us our most intense experience of an overwhelming sensation of pleasure and has thus furnished us with a pattern for our search for happiness." But Freud went on to say that repression of sexual urges is necessary to release energy for the development of civilization. If human beings let their sexuality run rampant, so Freud thought, civil life would collapse. Many major religions preach the same message, and sexual activity is rigorously controlled by family, church, and state all over the world.

How does sex fit into the philosopher's diet? Essentially, but with a light touch, I hope. Like Freud, I'll ask you to try to use some of that obsessive sexual energy to control your life. You've already learned to control your own sexual urges. On the other hand, like Henry Miller (whose books I read when they still had to be smuggled from Paris), I think Freud over-estimates the danger of hopping in bed when you get a good chance. It isn't civilization that free love might destroy, but merely prudish Victorian puritanism and the market economy in sex.

No, I've not answered the philosophical question. I'll use my sidle-up approach and make a few attempts. Sex is the sort of thing that may get you in trouble if you blurt right out what you have in mind.

When you think about sex, you have to think about the passions of love and hate; about power, exploitation, and the master-and-slave relations that Georg Wilhelm Friedrich Hegel in *Phenomenology of Spirit* and Jean-Paul Sartre in *Being and Nothingness* say are central in human affairs. You see, that is another trouble with the philosophy of sex. There is a great deal that is ludicrous and fun about human sexual engagements, but when you start trying to be philosophical about it, it gets *heavy*. Let me end this apologetic introduction to my chapter on sex by returning to Henry Miller. The form of *Tropic of Cancer* is a ribald, sexist, irreverent celebration of human sexuality. Its content reduces to: don't let them get you in their bag. That is: control your own life. In *The Books in My Life*, Henry Miller paid homage to the writers who influenced him, and now I want to acknowledge his influence on me.

Here is to Henry Miller, who made an advocate of free love out of a teenaged boy destined to go to Iowa State College of Agriculture and Mechanic Arts, where girls (including his future wife) had to be in their dormitories by 8:30 weeknights and 10:30 P.M. Saturdays. But you know, it didn't matter.

Henry Miller's is not the only inspirational literature about sex. There is almost nothing we don't know now about human sexual mechanics and physiology. Masters and Johnson, who attached electrodes to every possible orifice and protrusion to do the impeccable and indispensable scientific groundwork in this field, are from my university. A few years ago it was very in for an academic couple from Washington University to exhibit casually on their coffee table a copy of Masters and Johnson's *Human Sexual Response* with the inscription inside, "Thanks for your cooperation," signed, "Bill & Virginia."

I am skeptical of authors who tell you that you can use up calories by indulging in sexual activity. Most sexual liaisons are, after all, consummated in bed, which is not a very large arena for running around in. Perhaps you can use up a few calories by doing preparatory exercises beforehand, but sexercise books promising to set you up for the big scene are merely exercise books the publisher hopes you will buy because of your obsession with sex. They are just as good or bad as any other exercise book. But none of the sexercise books — even the ones that show you how to put what where and when — describes any activity that could get your heartbeat up above 125 for thirty or thirty-five minutes at a time. Of course, anybody can think of ways you could accomplish this in the sexual act, bu would it be fun to keep up that frantic a romp for thirty-five minutes? Running is one thing, but this is ridiculous.

There is much to say about sex, all of it relevant to the theme of this book. Let's begin with the fact that we all desire sexual satisfaction in the arms of someone who really turns us on. Do we have good examples of what turns us on? Of course. Turn to the centerfolds in *Playboy* and *Playgirl*. Here is your exercise: calculate the weight and height of the beautiful bodies displayed front center. Now turn to the advertisements in *Vogue* and the *New Yorker* and do the same for their models. See what I mean? The nude bodies we like to look at are inevitably shorter and heavier than the clothed bodies we like to look at. Almost all the nudes exhibited in the centerfolds exceed the average American weight for their height. A fair number of the men don't have much fat on them, but rise above average because of heavy muscles. As for the women, their excess can certainly be described clinically as fat, but it is seldom referred to in derogatory terms.

Now imagine the *Vogue* models without clothes. Look at those collapsed cheeks, the nonexistent calves, the bony hips. Long and tall, with sharp elbows and knees, men and women asexually alike.

This demonstrates again that being "overweight in America" is mostly a faddish figment of mind. When it comes to sexual desirability, contenders on the upper end of the weight scale for average Americans have the edge. In our sexual fantasies and in the flesh, we prefer someone with a little fat on his or her bones. This is shown by the way products are sold with sexy advertisements. Look at those rugged, big-thighed men and women in Marlboro ads. The American tobacco industry appeals to sexual preferences to sell cigarettes. Undress those big smokers and you have centerfolds.

Could thin models with hollow cheeks be used in cigarette advertising? Not to sell cigarettes to men who are worried about cancer. But cadaverous women in elegant clothes are used to sell Virginia Slims to women, who would like to look like the models.

This allows me to make a fine little philosophical point about knowledge and belief. You can perfectly well believe contradictory things, for example, that you can cheat on your diet and still lose weight. But you cannot *know* contradictory things, because knowledge must be consistent. Women know, for example, that size 12 bought off the rack at Penney's is considerably smaller than size 12 in expensive clothes. If you have been economical in buying your clothes but want to reduce your dress size, all you have to do is pay for it. You can know this, do this, and still believe you've lost weight. Bathroom scales are notoriously inaccurate, anyway.

It would be nice to wear those great clothes; on the other hand, do you want to look emaciated when you undress for a lover? This ambiguity perpetuates and feeds the diet industry. As long as we keep going up and down, the world will turn.

Yes, I know that sex is a serious matter. Like running, it is also another world. All we need discuss here is what will advance our program of taking weight off and keeping it off. Let's consider first the pleasure and use of anticipation, and then the relation of sexual satisfaction to the need for food.

One of the greatest success stories in the diet literature is that of Fats Goldberg of New York City. By the time Goldberg was twenty-five years old, he had weighed over 300 pounds for years. For many reasons he decided to lose weight, but most of them can be summed up in one word: girls. Not to put too fine a point on it, Fats wanted to get laid. I've never met Mr. Goldberg, but I like him. He went right to the heart of the matter. He didn't say that he just wanted to look better or be more fit, it wasn't mere vanity or health he had in mind; no, Fats Goldberg exposed his human soul. He wanted to love and be loved. Nobody loves a fat man. So Fats took it off and keeps it off.

How did he do it? For one thing, he knew what he wanted. There is nothing like the promise of paradise to get someone's attention. Anticipation is wonderfully mind-concentrating. Fats exploited anticipation to get there, and he still uses anticipation to stay there.

You know that it is not actually true that the best part about sex is thinking about it, but there certainly is a lot of savor in anticipation. Fats Goldberg sticks to a severe diet for six days a week. Then one day a

week, he has an orgy. On orgy days he goes to deli-
catessens, ethnic food stores, or fine restaurants, but
more often than not, he pigs out on junk food. His
diet allows him to eat all he wants once a week, but
Fats does not really pack it in on his feast days the
way he did when he weighed over 300 pounds. You
have to have a big capacity to eat 10,000 calories at a
sitting, even when on moral holiday. Fats just can't
eat that much anymore.

What keeps Fats going during the days of famine is
anticipation. Like us all, he thinks about food a lot.
He knows he can't have the real thing all the time.
One has other things to do than eat. In idle moments,
what he does is (to piggyback on a biblical phrase
President Carter made popular in a *Playboy* interview)
commit pig-out in his heart. This keeps him on the
straight and narrow. Then, one day a week he lets
himself go. Plato tells of a man who felt an overwhelming desire to look at a pile of mutilated bodies
but at the same time was sickened by the very thought
of it. Finally he could hold out no longer, rushed over
to look, and said, "Feast you damnable eyes, feast."
Fats Goldberg has now weighed 145 pounds for nearly
thirty years. The 300-pound man he once was still
haunts him, so once a week Fats leads this ghost to
the trough and says, "Eat, you pig!"

I bow to the Fats Goldberg method, but I think it
too severe for anyone who has never weighed 300
pounds. What is important for you in the Fats Goldberg method is to recognize and use anticipation.

Anticipation is salt and pepper waiting for the fried egg of life. It makes your mouth water. You can wait. It is sweet pain to hold off when you know the feast is coming. The more elaborate your planning, and the further in the future the consummation of the plan (think of heaven), the greater the pleasure. My fantasy about eating a meal prepared by the best chef in Lyon is a pornographic orgy of anticipation. You might have to save money for years before you could enjoy that meal. It would be worth it, both for the food and for its contribution to your program of staying at the weight of your heart's desire.

Thank you, Fats Goldberg.

Sexual exercise *does* use up calories, and I heartily recommend it whether you want to lose weight or not. Nevertheless, it really would be hard — and take more time — to use up the calories in sexual congress that you can burn off in a four-mile run. You can trust me: if sex *were* enough, I'd be the first to tell you. I think we must also discount those theories in some of the more racy diet books that hanky panky will divert your attention from food. Human beings are not, after all, like cats and dogs, who chase around for days without eating. As many affairs are conducted in coffee shops and restaurants as in motel rooms.

David Hume studied human nature by using himself as a model. He thought his own nature was much like anyone else's, and he seldom hesitated to generalize from his own responses to theories about human nature. I feel the same way. You know that old Latin phrase?

> *Triste est omne animal post coitum, praeter*
> *mulierem gallumque.*
>
> All animals are sad after sexual intercourse,
> except human females and roosters.

I suppose the melancholic male who coined that aphorism was thinking of the fact that after a really satisfying encounter, roosters crow and women go to sleep. My own experience is that I always feel wide awake, happy, and hungry afterwards. My thoughts naturally turn to the refrigerator. After sex, all men eat. From what I can discern about David Hume, I'm sure he would agree.

What about the theory that lack of affection, love, and sexual satisfaction causes people to seek comfort in food? Don't frustrated people go out and buy chocolates, take them to bed, and eat every one? Isn't it a vicious feedback cycle? Jack eats and gets fat because he has no lover, and then no one loves him because he is so fat, so he eats more and gets fatter. What about Jill, who will not diet for fear that she could not find a lover even if she were thin? Wouldn't a lover help Jack and Jill?

Yes.

I venture to predict, however, that sexual satisfaction alone will not help these people much in taking weight off and keeping it off.

All right, what if we purposefully deprived people

of sexual satisfaction on the opposite theory that they would then lose their appetites? I don't like this suggestion. Babies, and even some adults, who are deprived of love and affection sometimes pine away and die. I doubt that there is any known case in which the lack of sexual satisfaction was the direct cause of death, but even if sexual abstention did lead infallibly to weight loss, would I recommend it? Are you kidding? (Anyway, how many fat priests and nuns do you know?)

I had better leave these theories to my brother, who intends to write his own fat book. For all I know, my sister may write one, too, now that I have.

As I've already remarked, years ago I wrote a sensational book titled *Sex and Revolution*, which, for various reasons (all wise) I never tried to publish. My general thesis was that sexual revolution could lead to world economic revolution. It seems to me to be a pretty silly idea now because the powers-that-be co-opted the sexual revolution just as they did the hippies and renegade road runners. The next thing you know the Feds will be legalizing marijuana.

What about smoking? A woman philosopher who prefers to remain nameless says that she once was fat, but she controls her weight now by smoking. "The Surgeon General Has Determined That Cigarette Smoking Is Dangerous to Your Health," I once told her. "Look," she said, "I have this oral fixation, see, and I don't want to get fat. Sucking my thumb is not socially acceptable for someone of my age and station in life, so I smoke." Smoking is indeed an effective way of losing and keeping off weight. If you smoke, you can even knock off the running routine. However, as the Surgeon General reminds us, serious health problems derive from smoking, so I don't advise it as a way of keeping trim, even though I admire the professor in question excessively.

In my book on sex and revolution, I promoted the idea that if the masses took control of their sex lives in defiance of family, church, and state — all of which enforce rigid, repressive rules concerning sexual conduct — they might then take control of the world. My concern was not with the content, but with the form of the matter. Revolution, after all, requires commitment and the ability to focus and act on one unitary thing through thick and thin.

With respect to the content, I had a theory. People can survive without sexual satisfaction, but people cannot live without food. It seemed to me that if enough people took control of their sexual lives and assured themselves sexual satisfaction that they don't even need, then perhaps they could be convinced to take control of the world's food production in order to distribute food to a billion undernourished and starving people. This decommoditization of food would disrupt the world's businesses, industries, and governments, so a world economic revolution would be required. All because people who had liberated themselves sexually would realize that having won one battle against the powers-that-be that had deprived them of full sexual satisfaction, they could also liberate food production, a matter of life and death.

Because of those heavy factors — love and hate and the emotional dynamite of human interactions — I'm not sure I could tell you how to liberate yourself sexually, as I've told you how to lose weight and keep it off. I'm quite sure, on the other hand, that I don't have the foggiest idea how to take over the world's food production and distribute it to the needy. Corporate power, the state, and civilization itself rose on the stores of food that were produced, withheld, and bought and sold when human beings first invented agriculture 10,000 years ago. For details about that, see *Man and Nature*, which I wrote with my wife, Patty Jo Watson, and did publish. Now you see me trying once again to plant the stubborn seeds of revolution.

If you eat less, if you eat fresh fruit and vegetables and whole grain and range-fed meat, you will be raising a cry against agribusiness and the processed-food industry that have an iron grip on the world's food production and distribution. Food is the foundation of all power over human beings, for every day every one of us must eat. Your cry will be one drop of water in the wide, wide ocean, but if there were enough dissenters, a tidal wave would sweep the world.

It is something to think about. I throw it in on the chance that it might inspire you to maintain your weight program. For those of you who don't want to change the world but only yourselves, I don't suppose the exposure of my plans for world conquest through proper diet will worry you much.

Comes the crunch. There you are on the bed, the two of you, knee to knee. What does it all mean? I don't know. Some philosophers argue that the question makes no sense and thus has no answer. Others, like Richard Rorty, suggest that the question is useful for keeping the conversation going, in the pragmatic hope that talk is the moral equivalent of war. I said that philosophy consists of getting questions right. What about the answers? The word *philosophy* means literally the passive love of knowledge, but philosophy is often characterized as the active search for truth. Alas, the danger of a discipline dedicated to seeking the truth is that some people will get the idea that they have found it.

Some years ago I told the philosopher Richard Rudner that I had been working on the philosophy of sex for fifteen years, and had managed in that length of time to write seven pages.

"I'll tell you, Doc," he said, "fifteen years is not long enough and seven pages are too many."

I wish he could have lived so I could hear what he would have said when I told him that the chapter on sex in my book was very difficult to get a grip on, and the shortest.

6
How to Live

You know that to take off 20 pounds and keep them off you must change your life. It may be the hardest thing you ever do. It seems such a trivial thing. What is more ludicrous than perfectly healthy Americans living off the fat of the richest land in the world, huffing along the jogging trail, discussing calories and trading diets? Almost none of them are particularly overweight by any standard that Mother Nature ever devised. Eat, my children, eat and multiply, that is what Mother Nature advises. And we do.

But the content of our quest — its substance, its matter — is not the important thing, is it? If it were merely a matter of following fads, of looking forward to each new diet book, and yo-yoing with the seasons, well, that would be entertaining. But there is more.

Not the content, but the form. You want a new life, and if one way of attaining it is to gain control of your weight, why not do it? One way is as good as another so long as no one gets hurt.

I am seldom at a loss for words in face-to-face rep-artee. When my mother asked me in all seriousness in her seventieth year, "What's it all for?" I instantly shot back, "If it wasn't fun, it's too late now." That might have been a cruel thing to say to some mothers, but mine is as tough as nails. "Umm," she replied, turning back to her book. It was a psychohistory of Richard Nixon, as I recall. She follows the American political scene the way some people follow football, and she knows all the players.

My students ask, "What does it all mean?" And I admit that I am often tempted to reply in the words of Mr. Natural, Robert Crumb's great underground-comics characterization of God, who when questioned about the meaning of the cosmos answers, "Don't mean sheeit!"

What "it" is for is the enjoyment of life, and what it means is what you make of it. In this book I offer you the fierce satisfaction of taking control of a small part of your own life. Losing weight and keeping it off in America is ideal for this purpose. Any serious attempt makes you realize how damnably difficult it is. To do it means facing such opponents as those Federal Government officials who recently canceled a U.S. Agriculture Department publication on nutrition titled "Food II" because "the government shouldn't be publishing advice on how to lose weight," even though "Food I" had been a best-seller and seven million people had written in for the sequel.

How should you live?

Have fun, but try not to hurt anyone.

I know perfectly well that that is a dumb thing to say. How can I sit here telling Americans to have fun when unemployment is probably twice what government admits, and when a third of the world's population is poverty-stricken, oppressed, and undernourished or starving?

Because we pass this way but once. If you don't enjoy it now, it will be too late. And if you *are* worried about world hunger, you can help — however slightly — by changing your eating habits in a way that calls attention to waste and disproportion in world food production and distribution. It may be no more than a token gesture, but symbolic action is necessary in changing the world, too.

How can we avoid hurting anyone? I had a colleague once who swore over his lunch of smoked clams that he was in no way responsible for the starving Chinese (the victims date the story). He would admit that it is just our good luck to be born in America. Is it moral to enjoy this good fortune? Are you immoral if you continue to enjoy any of the accidental advantages, if you do anything less than a saint in helping the unlucky? There certainly are relations between our abundance and their poverty, but isn't it a world that neither we nor they ever made?

Philosophers always shift the question. I don't know how to determine our moral duties given the established world framework of rich and poor, powerful and weak, advantaged and disadvantaged in which we live. Perhaps we are immoral in accepting what we did not design and apparently cannot change. I leave that to go to the shifted question: what is the source of moral courage in those who *do* work for change?

Descartes said that if people do not believe in God and an afterlife, there is no hope of imposing morality on mankind. Yes, he said mankind, and I agree with feminist philosophers that we ought to begin with the morality of men. On the other hand, I hope Descartes is wrong about the goad of morality, because it is very difficult in our modern world to believe that there is a God Who will reward the virtuous by sending them to heaven and punish the sinful by sending them to hell. I've already remarked, by the way, that if you *do* want to believe in God, start going to church as Pascal advises: follow the form and eventually belief in the content will follow.

If you believe in God already, please do not ask Him to help you with your weight program. I am quite serious. We are looking for the source of moral courage. It is in you. You must change your life on your own. I don't think that if you believe in God your calling on Him won't help you. If you have confidence in His support, calling on Him (whether or not He exists) will probably help. But we depend too much on Big Brother already, and my radical intent is to get people to depend on themselves. I agree with David Hume that if there is a God Who has created us, He has a lot of explaining to do. Hume also points out that although Pascal's method of depending on faith rather than reason works, no one denies that there are false gods, and I would worry about which one, if any, was The True One. Hume makes the chilling suggestion that God may be a Committee.

Your strength and moral courage must come from within. Don't look for outside help. Human beings are capable of setting and reaching goals themselves. Today, however, even small accomplishments may seem impossible because the modern world, with its divisions of labor and immense variety of diversions, its demands and delights, makes it difficult for people to do a single, unitary thing of any kind for very long. College professors are fortunate to have schedules that provide time for concentrating their minds. This is not true for many people in business, government, and industry. Rather than a guaranteed annual minimum income, my utopia would provide a guaranteed annual block of time for thinking. Still, it does not take a philosopher to figure out that the only way to get a grip on your own life is by taking hold.

To take hold you must make a commitment to do this one thing:

You must change your life.

Fantasizing about a new life must be the favorite daytime occupation of Americans. A divorce rate of 35 percent suggests that a lot of people make the attempt. We change jobs and living places frequently, moving from city to city. These changes often look big, but they seldom result in a structural change in a person's life

People get divorced and marry other people very much like the ones they just divorced. Most American houses and apartments, American cities, American jobs, and American people are alike. You can eat the same junk food coast to coast without ever having to get more than a hundred yards from a highway or your car. Many of these big changes don't change your inner self. Real changes are difficult.

Besides taking weight off and keeping it off, there are many other seemingly small things that are very difficult to do. For example, choosing friends. Most of us do not choose friends, they are given to us. They are the people we went to school with, our workmates, the neighbors. Almost always the near at hand. You may have almost nothing else in common. Of course, some of these become dear friends. My closest friend for the last twenty years was forced on me by an accident of circumstance (and me on him). One of our joys together is cataloging our differences and shuddering at the thought of how horrible it would be to live the other's life.

It would be cruel to keep count of friends who are useful and every year cross off those who are not, but you can still choose new friends who share your interests and enhance your life. It takes an effort. You must seek them out in their native habitats. You must also find out your own true nature. Trial and error is necessary for this. You might learn, for example, whether you really want to be a biologist — with biologists for friends — not merely by studying to be a biologist, but by finding out where biologists eat lunch and joining them. You might find that you prefer musicians.

This may seem obvious to you, as it is. But after many years of counseling students, I know that it is a serious, sometimes heartbreaking matter, and that it must be said over and over again. You *can* make your own choices. There is enormous pressure on you to take what you get. We are expected to make friends among those we are thrown with, the people who study or work or live where we do. It comes as a revelation to some people that they can choose their friends, their professions, their leisure activities. You can go out on your own.

The same goes for choosing a spouse. I once had an exasperated argument with a friend (with whom I've been having exasperated arguments for thirty-five years) who wanted to find a life's companion to sail around the world with him. "And you're looking in St. Louis, Missouri?" I asked. If you want to marry a ski bum, go to a ski resort. (Yes, I like things to be wrapped up, too. He is living with a woman now who is a good sailor, but he didn't find her in St. Louis, and he no longer wants to sail around the world.)

I'll tell you who changes their lives in America: middle-aged women. Their children are grown and gone from home, or their husbands have left them, or they left home themselves one Monday night and their husbands didn't even notice. Sometimes they take philosophy courses. They are not always the smartest students, but they are almost always the *best* students. They are changing their lives. I bow to these women just as I bow to Fats Goldberg.

Did I say it is difficult to change? For example, you might think it easy for college students to change their majors, or switch from one college to another. For many, these things are so hard to do as to be almost impossible. A student gets started in something somewhere, and that's it. I knew someone in college who is now a successful engineer. He hated engineering at the end of his first week in college, and he hated it when he graduated four years later near the top of his class. For all I know, he hates it still. It seems to me now that he went too far in ignoring content for the sake of form. He did get a lot of satisfaction from setting out to do something and doing it. Obviously I admire this, but wouldn't it be better to choose something you like to do?

I intend my program to offer more than mere satisfaction in having done a difficult thing. Still, it is the satisfaction in reaching one's goal that I am stressing. When very bright students, extremely accomplished in both the humanities and the sciences, come to me agonizing about what to do, I give them Descartes's advice. It does not matter whether you become an English professor or a physicist; but to become good in either you must choose one or the other. Choose one. It does not matter which; what matters is that you make the choice and stick to it. Don't look back. More recently this rule of behavior has become known as a self-fulfilling prophecy. But prophecy is not enough: you have to act on it. If you commit yourself to being a physicist now, fifteen years from now (remember Pascal) you will be a physicist. Probably you will be happy with what you are then. If not, well . . . you know what to do.

Suppose you have a clubfoot but want to be a ballet dancer? Suppose you find at the age of thirty-five that you really wanted to be a pianist rather than a dentist. It is impossible and it is too late. What about my simplistic advice for the forlorn then? Then I advise you to read Jean-Paul Sartre's *Being and Nothingness*. It is too hard? It is incredibly hard. If you can get through that book and really understand it, you'll have accomplished a very difficult task. Philosophy is no easier than life.

Did I take that advice myself in choice of friends, spouse, and career? Not always. Never mind what I do. While there is something in the claim (which Descartes also made) that you can learn more about a person by watching what he does than by listening to what he says, it is good for you to understand that it is better to follow what some people say (Descartes among them) than to imitate what they do. Descartes was one of the most boorish health nuts who ever lived. He was always telling his city friends how his quiet and measured country life had improved his health. Actually, it did.

If you are serious about losing weight and keeping it off, listen to what I say.

My program will give you rare delight.

But if you don't have fun doing this thing, my friend, then it will be the dumbest damned thing you have ever done. I don't mean taking weight off and keeping it off, I mean the crucial matter of gaining control of part of your life. *That's* what you'd better glory in; otherwise you might as well ask your mother what to do next.

Here is the sticker: you won't know if you enjoy it until you do it. To find out, you have to commit yourself to attaining the goal. You must take what Kierkegaard called a leap of faith. Of course Kierkegaard — like Pascal — worried about whether or not his choice of belief in Christianity was the right one. Do I dare compare a decision to go on a diet with a decision to become a Christian? Absolutely. You aren't choosing just to go on a diet, remember; you are changing your life.

My program is not so different from Pascal's, except in one crucial way. Pascal asks you to have faith in God and do what He commands. I ask you to have faith in yourself and do what you want. Do you want to change your life? Do you want to control your own life? Then do it.

You could also join the Navy and see the world. I am asking you to cast your lot in a game whose goal is diametrically opposed to that of the Army or the Air Force or the Marines. Military officers can teach you self-control. You can be trained, for example, to salivate at the sound of a bell like Pavlov's dog. Military training is calculated to make you loyal as a dog.

Unfortunately, for many, it is always the year and the day of the dog. Plato had a theory about it. He said that there are three kinds of people: rulers controlled by reason, soldiers and police controlled by willpower, and workers controlled by desire. He thought people were born as one or the other. Plato went on to say that the best soldiers and police are faithful dogs. They have immense loyalty and self-control and follow orders without thinking. In the ideal state, rulers were to use the soldiers and police to control the workers. The result was to be a harmonious society for the benefit of all.

You must understand that the kinks in this system are still being ironed out.

Plato also said that every individual has reason, willpower, and a set of desires. Each of us is dominated by one or another of the three. You must be satisfied with your lot because there is no way of altering the proportions with which you were born.

This is an excellent theory for ideological and propaganda purposes for rulers who want to keep people down on the farm, or in the factory or ghetto.

Reason, willpower, and desire. Well, why not? Descartes and Pascal thought much the same. You can derive comfort from knowing that you are a slob and a clod by nature and that it would be foolish to try to do anything about it. Boots of lords and empire builders have been licked since civilization began by people convinced that they were naturally inferior — good folk, but a little slow, whose lives have to be shaped for them for their own good.

This is also the gospel of the advertising industry. The theory is that almost everybody is so dumb that ways can be devised to sell anybody anything. Advertising geniuses are helped by loyal media personnel who are not asked to think but only to follow orders. And the meek will buy the earth. At the very least, the masses are convinced to buy white bread and sugar-loaded processed foods of every sort. The ideal advertising target is a little child. Have you watched any children's television programs recently?

Like anyone who makes a living teaching, I very much suspect that most people — particularly children and teenagers — are a lot smarter than they let on. (Kenneth Grahame wrote in *The Golden Age* about "monkeys, who very sensibly refrain from speech, lest they should be set to earn their livings.") Still, the advertising industry is one force that makes it awfully hard for you to take off 20 pounds and keep them off.

Most behavior-modification techniques being developed and used in the world today are for the purpose of modifying others. He who does the modifying thereby gains great power and control. Even when changes are made with therapeutic techniques designed to increase a patient's self-control, it is always difficult for the patient to leave the therapist, and the relapse rate is high.

I'm providing you with a method of changing your own behavior. I want you to be intensely aware of who is in charge. Self-control is *you* in control. You must do the work. I'm willing to be your coach, but I don't want to be your leader. Is this something a person has to be predisposed to before he or she can do it? Sure, but that's a self-fulfilling prophecy. Go to it. I'll tell you how to do it. If you do it, you have to do it on your own. Go on, now. There are some things we can do only for ourselves. Don't depend on me, do it yourself. Nobody is coercing you. Nobody else can do it for you. I might cheer if you win, but that's because I have a natural tendency to get carried away at sporting contests. I can't take any credit. I can lead a horse to water, but I can't make it drink.

OK, OK, OK.

But listen: don't form a club of graduates of the program. If you need that kind of back slapping, you've not yet made it.

Let me tell you a story. One of the greatest characters of seventeenth-century France was a man named Desbarreaux. Once when asked what his profession was, he replied, "Seeking good wine by land and by sea." He moved from place to place according to season, eating the finest delicacies of Europe. He was also much in demand as a conversationalist. One year he set out with a friend on a quest for truth. His friend carefully avoided taking Desbarreaux through the fabled vineyards of Languedoc, for Desbarreaux had a tendency to believe that having found good wine he had found truth. They could not have found truth in Languedoc, for Descartes was in Holland, and to visit him was their goal.

Descartes greeted them with open arms. The three boon companions are the models for the characters in the only dialogue Descartes ever wrote. His friend Desbarreaux is represented as an intelligent layman whose instinctive good sense approves the truths of Cartesianism. The next two paragraphs are also part of the story, so don't be confused.

People expect so much of philosophers. It is a little ridiculous, especially today when so much of professional philosophy is involved in working out intricate problems that require several years of coursework in philosophy to understand and great analytic skills to solve. To tell the truth, a philosopher is just about the last person I would go to for practical advice.

But then I never claimed that my program for taking off weight and keeping it off was practical, did I? I claim merely that it will work. And that it won't hurt anybody. And that you can do it if you will.

Back to Descartes's chateau. After six months, Desbarreaux had the greatest praise for the food and wine of Holland. It was Descartes's cook who prepared the food, and the wine came from Descartes's cellar. The moral of the story is: you can trust a philosopher to select good food and wine.

How to live? With as much enjoyment as possible without hurting others. Of course, there will be pain and misery in your life. Inevitably you will hurt others. See how my train of thought goes? We Americans are extremely fortunate to be able to enjoy the bounty of this great land. Again, do we deserve it? I don't think so, but the question may be impossible to answer. Certainly we have no right to ignore or scorn the unfortunate. Some of the things we do without thought increase their misery.

Because this is a book of truth telling, we must face the fact that not many Americans are going to do anything about decreasing the world's hunger. I have tried to provide some inspiration for those of you who care. If you follow this program, you will be hungry much of the time for a year or so until you adjust to your maintenance diet. It won't hurt you, but your body will take a long time to adapt to the change of food and lowered caloric intake. Perhaps you will fast for a day or two now and then to make up for binges. By doing this you will have a gut comprehension of what hunger really is for as many as a third of the world's people. Perhaps it will make you think.

Then there is the matter of going off sugar, white flour, and other processed foods. When I was a child living in a small town in Iowa, my father, who was superintendent of the local primary and secondary schools, entertained himself by keeping a cow and a pig and by raising a garden. (Of course, we bought sugar and white flour. How else could my mother be a world-class cake baker?) Almost everyone living in small towns across America still has a garden. In many parts of the world, it is possible to raise a large proportion of one's annual food in home gardens. If you keep a cow and a pig, so much the better. (I recommend a Jersey cow, by the way. You may never have tasted Jersey milk and cream and butter. Butter that you have churned yourself. Yes, you would have to learn how to milk a cow. Won't you please recognize nostalgia when you see it? And note that *Jersey* is not a trademark but a kind of cow. Jersey cows have the sweetest faces of any four-footed animal alive.)

Gardening is another world. You don't need a very large piece of ground to plant a garden. Yes, I know we are a nation mostly of city dwellers, so you cannot be expected to raise your own food. Modern civilization depends on the many subsisting on food raised by the few. If we are not all to be self-subsistent farmers, then we have to depend on others to produce food, just as many small nations cannot produce everything they need to be part of the modern world, but often must concentrate on one crop or resource for export.

I'm coming to processed foods. As the philosopher J. L. Austin says, "There's the bit where you say it and the bit where you take it back." I am now at the crucial juncture. You can go off processed foods entirely for six months or a year. Fanaticism can carry you that far. If you are careful, you can avoid a lot of sugar and white flour the rest of your life. But the fact is that unless you join a natural-food commune — and you might — you can't avoid all commercial processed foods. Notice the "commercial." Even my father pro-

cessed our food for winter. He butchered and preserved meat and he bottled grape juice and tomato
juice. (When my father retired, I suggested that he
increase the size of his garden and put up food that I
would buy for my winter supplies. "Are you crazy?"
he said. "We haven't canned anything for years." Well,
he *did* still put peas and berries in a big freezer. He
wasn't about to put any up for me. "You can buy it
at the store," he said. Which reminded me then as it
reminds me now that about six weeks after I started
college, my father sold the cow. I'd been milking it
morning and night since I was twelve, and after I left
home, my father soon decided that there was no reason
to get up every morning to milk a cow when you could
buy milk and butter at the store.)

You understand that I'm trying to get you to buy a
cow, don't you? Where I came from, you say to someone who has taken on a long-term daily commitment,
"Bought a cow, did you?"

They didn't use the additives and preservatives back
in those days that commercial processors do today, but
semantic quibbling over the word *processed* is not the
point. I want to take you over the watershed.

Lovely kosher dill pickles.

You get the point. I really hope you will avoid snacks
made out of salt and plastic; "ice cream" spun out of
sugar, oil, and air; meat full of preservatives, hormones, and antibiotics. You have to eat some processed
foods. But read the labels, pick and choose. OK? The

trick is that philosophers never really take it all back. They know you'll remember the part where they said it, making it impossible for you to get it all back.

You see, I *do* know you can't keep a pig in your condominium.

Let's go on to something else.

I keep talking of worlds and games, so I want to explain what I mean. You may have become convinced that the author of this book is a fanatic. This is, as philosophers always say and as I've said before, in a sense true. The sense in which it is true is that I urge you to undertake one major activity unified by a single goal. You can lose 20 pounds and keep them off. You know by now that the weight program is the content, fanatical commitment the form. As a philosopher, I am most interested in the exercise as one of developing and imposing one's free will. Self-control, that's the general form of the game. The general content is life. Let's get on with it.

Having nearly finished this book without looking at what's new in the field, I went down to the Stanford University Bookstore to see if there was anything new I should read in the fat-book line.

The Stanford University Bookstore has a marvelous collection of diet, health, nutrition, food, behavior-modification, and exercise books. Oddly enough, they need beefing up in the running section, which seems peculiar to me because the largest publisher of running books — World Books — has its offices only about five miles from the bookstore.

Was there anything new in the fat-book line? Sure, lots, but nothing really new. I did buy and read a couple of them, though. Everybody needs inspirational reading.

Let me say something more about reading. I have already suggested that you read the diet, cookbook, health, and running literature for inspiration. You are reading an inspirational book now. I don't recommend those weight programs that involve your contracting with a lover to control your food intake, or pledging with Overeaters Anonymous, or joining Weight Watchers. There is even a blackmail program now in which you can contract with someone to deprive you of the necessities of life if you don't stay on your diet. These programs may work, but I don't recommend them because they all depend on other people. That isn't the name of the game in this book, is it? Any reduction and maintenance technique that requires the support of someone else (even God) is not going to result in your taking off weight and keeping it off *on your own*. Sure, you can put on a collar and have someone lead you to and from the table on a leash. But is it really true that we are either masters or slaves, as Hegel and Sartre suggest? There is certainly a lot of evidence that people do get caught in a master/slave world. It's not a game I'm interested in playing, either as master or as slave. I love to give advice, but I expect you to think it over and make your own choice. Plato was really off his rocker when he suggested that philosophers should be in charge. As a matter of fact, one of Plato's students — the tyrant Dionysius — did become a ruler and called Plato in to help. It's a long story, but the punch line is that things went to hell, Plato got sold into slavery, and his friends had to buy him back. There are masters and slaves.

I was talking about reading. You can read a book anywhere, anytime, alone. It is a matter between you and the author. I don't say that a book might not become your master, but you are free to read it over and over again. You can get on top of a book and either agree with it, or break its back.

Reading opens new worlds. John Stuart Mill thought that if only the masses would learn to read, they could change the world. It didn't turn out to be quite that simple, but reading how is the first step. (Note that censorship is a frontline defense in totalitarian regimes.)

I said that how to live is with as much enjoyment as possible. Whatever the prospects after death, this is the only life you will ever have. My mother wondered why she and my father had done all those things over the years — officiating, housekeeping, entertaining, participating. My father taught history and algebra while being superintendent and coach (it was a very small town) for forty-five years. He directed the senior class play. My mother helped him with everything. My father and mother worked for school and community almost every day and night of the week. Well, they enjoyed it. I was there long enough to know.

My mother wonders what it might have been like had she or my father made another choice. What if both of them had become lawyers? They would have been good ones. They could have gone into politics. My mother would have liked that. They made a choice and it structured their lives. It was all right even if my mother does wonder about it.

What about you? You are probably dissatisfied with some part of your life. How about restructuring it? Did I say that it isn't easy to change your life, even in such a simple matter as taking off weight and keeping it off? It can be done. You have to concentrate on something, make a commitment, and do it. You can do it if you want to. And enjoy it.

If you can't live it, read about it. That's what my mother does. And try not to hurt anyone.

7

How to Die

I N the dark of the cave, we had come to the pit we
had to cross. The three of us crouched in an opening
the size of a picture window, peering twenty feet across
to the passage that continued on the other side. The
light from our carbide lamps did not reach the bottom,
but we tossed in rocks to guess that the pit was maybe
fifty feet deep. No one had been down it. No one had
been very far along the passage across it. We were
exploring.

Bill was having trouble with his lamp, so he sat down
behind us in the passage to work on it. Dave started
across the pit while I stayed in the window watching.
Halfway across the pit Dave's body overbalanced. He
fell slowly away from the wall, turned completely over
in the light of my lamp, and disappeared into silent
blackness. He didn't say a word. Eons later there was
a quiet thud.

I had been told by the first explorers that there was
a crack in the floor of the passage on the other side

that might lead to the bottom of the pit, but I was across the pit and had shinnied twenty-five feet down the crack before I knew what I was doing. All the while I was yelling to Dave that everything would be all right. I didn't believe a word of it. I knew that my old friend was dead.

The last ten feet to the bottom of the pit seemed to be sheer, smooth limestone wall. As I reached it I heard Dave groan. Unbelieving, I just let go and slid the rest of the way down.

He lay on a thirty-degree slope of mud with his head pointing down. He had fallen flush on the slope between two large pointed boulders and had slid down until his head was just at the edge of a deep pool of water. He was bleeding from a cut where his hard hat had smashed against his ear, but there seemed to be no broken bones. "I'm all right," he said, and stood up. We figured out how to climb the wall, met Bill on his way down, and the three of us crossed the pit at the top again. That was enough exploring for one day. Four hours later we were outside.

On another trip into the cave, we measured Dave's fall: forty-four feet.

After that fall Dave and I continued to explore caves for many years. Or I should say that we continued to explore a cave, for we were in the Flint Ridge Cave System in Kentucky, then the second-longest known cave in the world. We were trying to climb the Everest of world speleology. Our quest was to connect the Flint Ridge Cave System with Mammoth Cave, the third-longest in the world. (The longest was Hölloch in Switzerland.) If we made the connection, the resulting system would become the longest cave in the world. We worked on it weekends, holidays, and summers for twenty years before the connection was made. Roger Brucker and I wrote a book about it: *The Longest Cave.* At the time the connection was made, the only active explorers who had stayed with it for the entire time were Roger and I. Neither of us was a member of the final party that made the connection.

There were other incidents like Dave's fall, but of the several hundred serious cavers who explored and mapped the 144 miles of cave passages in that cave system during those twenty years, not one was badly injured or killed. I have often wondered why not. Caving is basically underground mountaineering on muddy rocks in the dark, and in Flint Ridge you are taking the chance of being killed. You accept the odds.

Why?

Because exploring the great cave — learning the skills that few others possess and going places where no other human being has been and where few others will follow — is something that fills your soul with everlasting joy and with memories that nothing but total senility or death can ever efface.

All it required was total commitment for a few years, or perhaps, if you slipped once too often, for a lifetime.

I don't suppose many of you want to explore a big cave or climb a high mountain or sail around the world

These are adventures to read about, though. There ought to be something *you* can do that is as satisfying and doesn't require highly specialized skills or putting your life in danger.

I'm talking about form.

The crucial thing is commitment. And the content does matter. It seems to me that jogging is popular because it's so simple. You can run anywhere. Unlike football, baseball, tennis, or even skiing, the difference between what you are doing and what the world-class runners do is not all that great. To improve your status, all you have to do is move down the road a little faster.

I want to compare here the commitment involved in someone who decides to climb Everest with the commitment required to lose 20 pounds and keep them off. The words seem almost tangible as I search for just the right ones so this transition does not appear to be grotesque, ludicrous, and absurd.

Reinhold Messner and Peter Habler were the first two human beings to climb Everest without oxygen. Messner thereafter continued to push himself to the limits of his, indeed to the limits of human, capacity. A few years later he became the first human being ever to climb Everest without oxygen, *alone*.

Absolutely incredible.

And Messner is still pushing.

"He'll cash in one of these days," a friend said to me.

"Of course," I replied. "He knows it."

Is it right to commit yourself to an activity in which you know the end result will be death? Of course it is. It is, after all, right to commit yourself to life.

If you would like to do one difficult thing in your life that requires total commitment, something that if accomplished would fill you with joy and satisfaction for the rest of your life, then the content matters, but it is the form that carries you through, the form that counts.

As for content, there are two rules: whatever you do, try to have fun doing it. And try not to hurt anyone.

Losing 20 pounds and keeping them off for the rest of your life is as good a content as many. Don't knock it. Don't let other people knock it. It doesn't put you out there on the edge of the cliff where one false step means oblivion, but in some ways it is harder than exploring big caves and climbing high mountains. The weight game is not one that lasts for only a few years, after which you can retire gracefully with your laurels and get fat. It lasts a lifetime . . . and there are no laurels.

What about Messner and those like him who push it until they peel off a wall? This chapter is, after all, about how to die. My answer, as you can guess, is that you should endeavor if at all possible to die with class. People pushing limits, like Messner, have at least the satisfaction of knowing that if they die in the act, it will be in good form.

Suicide? Don't be absurd. They don't want to die.

They don't intend to die. They choose to do something very difficult right at the limits of human possibility in order to savor the joy and satisfaction of having done it. The risk is essential. It defines how hard it is. Even more, risk of death raises awareness of life to a peak. Socrates said, Know thyself. On the edge we are reminded of our mortality, knowledge of which makes us human.

I'm afraid that the fun of exciting, risky games also leads us to war. There are individual skills involved in fighting, but when you take as your adversary another human being rather than a mountain or a cave, you have hit upon an instance when content changes the form of the game. Mine is a game of self-control and self-reliance. In war you abandon yourself to those who order you to kill. I ask you to be fanatical about leading your own life. In war, fanatics forget themselves to follow a leader — and everyone gets hurt.

While writing this book, I have thought many times of the philosopher Richard Rudner. He was the chairman of my department and I think he hired me in part because it amused him to call me Doc Watson.

On sabbatical in the south of France, Rudner became aware of a severe pain in his back. Local doctors could not diagnose it, and since our home university has as good a medical school as any in the world, Rudner flew to St. Louis to have a checkup. He was told that he had cancer throughout his body, and that if it were not arrested, he had about three months to live.

They gave him chemotherapy, which inhibits the growth and division of cancer cells. Unfortunately, it does the same for white blood corpuscles that fight infection. Rudner lasted six weeks before he caught a blood infection and died. He was fifty-seven.

This led to the following exchange. A good friend was lamenting how Rudner had died in full middle age.

"Middle age?" the wag he was talking to said. "Jerome, no one lives to be a hundred and fourteen."

Rudner would have loved that crack. It was made by one of his old students. Only a couple of years later that student himself died of cancer at the age of forty-seven. Both he and Rudner would have appreciated the irony.

Rudner died in elegant form. He was working on a book and was corresponding with other philosophers. In great pain and nausea, he continued to put his papers together, to wrap things up in preparation for the inevitable. He fought like hell to continue the life he enjoyed so much. He remained the village atheist to the end and expected nothing beyond.

A few hours before he died, he told his family he would see them tomorrow. He didn't.

I know that one of Richard Rudner's greatest anguishes before he died was that he had not completed the book he had been working on for many years. Of course, he was anguished at not being able to grow old with the woman he loved, at not being able to see his grandchildren. But I think he would sigh tolerantly and approve of the point I'm going to make of his story; and he would have said with that pained look on his face he got whenever I piled pomposity on platitude, "You tell 'em, Doc." It is this:

Write your book before you die.

To write is to die a little. It is a good way to go. It is like having children. You created them, but once they go their own way, there is nothing much you can do about it. Sometimes it is nice to think that they will still be yapping away, after you yourself are gone.

Write your book before you die. You will get great satisfaction from it.

That's the form of the thing. The content is any serious expression of self that does not harm others. It takes some dedication, some commitment. It is taking control of part of your life to shape it as you will.

For those philosophers who think that mind and body are identical, that matter is all that exists, my program ought to be a piece of cake. Its content, however, may not appeal to them. Some of the best philosophers are fat.

Let me tell you how David Hume died. I have already told you that in his youth he was a lean, hawkish fellow who began to eat himself silly after undergoing an extreme intellectual crisis during which he despaired of ever finding truth. He never found truth, but he was a fat, jolly fellow the rest of his life, and a champion player of whist. He once said that in ordinary life one should exercise clever prudence and common sense. Philosophy should be done only in one's closet. There is no question in my mind that when he said this he winked broadly to his card companions and made an exaggerated gesture with his chin in the direction of the W.C.

The French bluestocking ladies loved Hume and called him *le bon David*. *Le grand bon vivant, David Hume.* What he died of was probably stomach cancer, which gripped his gut and wasted him away. He took it in good grace, encouraged his friends to visit him in his sickroom, and told them to cheer up.

The reports of Hume's good spirits and demeanor much disturbed another of the great characters of the eighteenth century, James Boswell, the famous biographer of Dr. Johnson. Boswell was disturbed because Hume was a notorious atheist, and it was not right that an atheist should go cheerfully to his doom. Boswell himself was a Christian, and a believer, who greatly feared for the salvation of his own soul because of his weaknesses for lying and whoring. He could not rest until he saw Hume.

Who knows how Hume felt physically on the day of Boswell's descent? It surely did not matter. *Le bon David* knew why Boswell was there, and he rose to the occasion. Never had he been so gay, so witty, so droll. He parried Boswell's every probe; and with every cheerful quip, he sank Boswell's hopes for heaven farther toward the depths of hell. Boswell went home in such a state of depression that he himself took to bed. And lo, he had a dream. He dreamed that Hume had recanted and confessed, and had died in the arms of

Jesus. It wasn't true, of course, but Boswell could not bear thinking of the alternative.

David Hume died in excellent form.

After a funeral you have a big meal. Food and fat are not just symbols of life, they sustain it. To deny them is to deny a little bit of life. If you take off 20 pounds and keep them off, you will often be reminded of the way it must be in the end.

I'm not sure how you are going to weather this heavy writing. We have already been through the hellfire and brimstone chapter. This is the chapter in which you find out for whom the bell tolls.

What I have to say is that fat, my friends, is in my book a metaphor. Fat represents the nagging triviality, the utter banality, and the inevitability of ordinary reality that separate us from what we think we want to be. It is the fleshly part of ourselves that binds us to this earth and keeps us from eternal life. My thesis is that the myth of heavenly paradise is but a dream of attenuated earthly joys abstracted from the trials and tribulations of daily life.

Render out some of that fat. Get down to the muscle. Bare yourself to the rising wind. I have said before and I will say again that it really does not matter much to the rest of us what you do, so long as you don't hurt anyone. But if you don't do something you will be proud of later on, it will matter to *you*.

Take hold and fight.

You can do it even if your father was not Scot, nor your mother Welsh.

My father starved to death in his eighty-first year of life. "Mark nineteen eighty," he said. "It's a bad year." It was for him.

The Omaha surgeons disagreed on what went wrong in his gut. There was a tumor, but evidently not a malignant one. After the tumor was removed adhesions closed his bowels. Another operation. Then adhesions blocked the kidneys. Another operation. They finally got a straight shot through his gut, but he had had it. "Let's get out of this place and go home," he said.

Instead of going home, we moved him to a small community hospital five miles from the school in which he had taught most of his life. Everyone there knew him. One of the nurses was the daughter and granddaughter of two women who had graduated from the high school when my father was superintendent. He still needed a lot of care and he knew it. At least he was close to home.

When my father was settled in his bed, he said to the doctor, "I don't want any more of those goddamned tubes down my nose or needles in my arm." They glared at each other. They had known each other for forty years, two dominating and authoritative men in that small, rural Iowa community, used to being looked up to, used to being obeyed.

The doctor looked down and said, "You know what that means, Prof."

My father said nothing, but nodded with grim satisfaction; when the doctor turned to me, I shrugged my shoulders, and he walked out.

I spent the last three weeks of his life with my father. When I arrived, he called me over and said, "Now Dick, I'm dying. Don't give me any crap that I'm not."

"OK, so you're dying. Now what?" I said.

He just closed his eyes and grinned.

His mind was, as they say about those who die from eating the Destroying Angel mushroom, clear to the last.

A few days before he died, a favorite niece and her husband visited him. As they got up to go, the husband said, "Now Prof, I want you to be sitting up in a chair next time I see you."

My father reared up in bed with the old diabolical leer in his eyes and said, "You don't see too many people buried sitting up, Giles."

I tried to feed him and he tried to eat. He could get a little down, and it went on through. But it wasn't enough.

He gagged. He hated the mashed chicken. "Chicken feathers," he would say when I would sneak in a bite. "I don't want any more of those damned chicken feathers." He would drink a bit of chocolate milk.

One late afternoon, in the last slanting light of a winter's day, my father asked me to help him turn over on his side. I did and said, "Is that better?"

"Hell no, it isn't better," he said. "You always did ask the dumbest questions."

I sat back down with my book.

In a little while he said, "It's all right."

About fifteen minutes later I noticed that he had quit breathing.

Here are some things my father loved to eat. Bread and milk. The bread was fresh out of the oven, grainy and moist, the hard, shiny crust scented with lard that had been smeared on it for glazing. The milk was fresh and warm from his old Jersey cow. My father liked a thick slice of bread, and he did not break it up. He folded it once and shoved it whole into the glass of milk, then smashed it down and ate it with a spoon. When I was a child I would watch him, and sometimes he drooled on purpose and rolled his eyes. "Watson, stop that," my mother would say.

My father liked to take a big chunk of butter churned from the cream of his old Jersey cow, put it on a bare plate, pour sorghum molasses on it, and smash the mess up into foam with a fork. Then he would spread the whole onto a thick slice of bread. The molasses crusted, the butter cut its sweetness, and the taste was like ambrosia.

My father liked Missouri Wonder beans — not your common Kentucky Wonder bean, he would say, but the Missouri Wonder that he had brought with him when he moved north to Iowa in 1922. He liked a fresh pan of beans to be half green pods and half shelled, boiled with a lot of small chunks of bacon. He would eat this with shining white slices from a raw winter onion as large as an apple. Hot beans, salty bacon, and cold, sweet onion. Never did a man eat so good.

My father grew tomatoes, which he sliced and ate raw with salt. He bottled thick tomato juice for winter. He liked to put several spoons of sugar into a glass of tomato juice, drink the juice down an inch or two, then fill the glass to the top again by adding milk. Stir. Drink.

My father raised four kinds of grapes; three kinds of apples; peaches; and plums. He raised strawberries, black and red raspberries, blackberries, boysenberries, gooseberries, and currants. Rhubarb, kohlrabi, and popcorn.

My mother made jelly from the black raspberries, and my father liked to spread thick, yellow butter and great globs of black-raspberry jelly on his bread. The gooseberries were for gooseberry pie. The rhubarb was boiled thick and eaten with much sugar and cream. He liked to eat the kohlrabi peeled and raw. He popped popcorn and poured so much melted butter on it that your fingers grew slippery while eating it.

My father hunted and fished all his life. He liked catfish dipped in cornmeal batter and fried in deep lard. He liked squirrel gravy.

My mother made noodles and cooked them with pot roast. She fried chicken. She baked bread. She fed my father.

My father liked . . . he liked to eat. I don't know what he liked best of all. Probably bread and milk.

That was what he asked for most during the final days of his life. But maybe what he liked best was gravy made from ham grease mixed with cream. He would take a thick slice of bread and put it on his plate, and spoon on ham gravy until all the bread was soaked through. The thin gravy ran all over the plate. My father would eat the soaked bread quickly, then mop up the rest of the gravy with more bread. I can see him now, hunched over his plate, jerking his chin up sharply to catch some gravy running down and threatening to drip on his shirt. He grins at the small boy across the table and takes another bite.

"Oh, Watson, stop that," my mother says, and my father's joy is complete.

Conclusion

L ET's get on with it.
I urge you to live at the peak of enjoyment of
life. Descartes said that the essence of the soul is self-
consciousness. If you want to enjoy your life, pay
attention to what you are doing. Control as much of
your life as you can. Live in full consciousness. And
don't stop thinking for yourself. If you don't think for
yourself, you will be someone's slave. Or dead.

Yes, there are masters and slaves. Descartes thought
there were also two other kinds of people: those concerned with learning things and those concerned with
making money. This dichotomy has been remarkably
persistent among philosophers who have tried to understand human nature and society. The dividing line —
like that between life and death — is apparently a knife's
edge. There are those who seek knowledge and those
who seek power, dreamers and merchants, professors
and politicians. Of course, some philosophers have
beaten their pens into swords, but on the whole, phi-

losophers write books rather than sign orders of exile and execution.

For those of you who read the conclusion first, let me remark that you may find my voice a bit heavy here and there, and feel as though I sometimes run along ahead, looking back at you and thumbing my nose. But remember what we are about. My father was a high school coach and he wanted me to be an engineer. This book is not only for my living mother, it is also for my dead father. I believe he died at peace.

It is true, of course, that while I don't think many people will actually follow my diet program, I do hope that most of you will enjoy reading my book. As for benefit, who is to say? For those few of you who choose to take off weight and keep it off and carry on, rest assured. You can do it if you will. If not, *c'est la vie*.

I am fifty years old, 5'8" tall, and weigh 150 pounds. I reached my present height and weight when I was sixteen and held there into my early twenties. Since then I have gone up and down from 140 to 170 pounds several times, and have held strong at 150 to 160 for many a year. My daughter and I stuck religiously to the program for about a year and a half, several years ago. It served its purpose, and incidentally taught me how to keep my weight closer to 150 than to 170. I do not think those 20 pounds make any serious difference to my health or well-being at all. If I keep at 150 it is merely as an exercise of my will and my conceit.

I knew you would want to know those things in that

last paragraph. You already know about my family.

It is always nice to close a book with a thought from Descartes, the father of modern philosophy. Descartes was also the father of an illegitimate daughter, the small Francine. He loved her dearly. When Francine was five years old, she came down with scarlet fever. In a dispassionate letter, Descartes reported that she suffered three days, turned purple, and died.

Descartes was devastated, and he cried like a baby. This was to his credit, one might say, but Descartes prided himself on being a pious man and so was vulnerable to criticism. Thus, a minister of the gospel publicly chastised Descartes for falling by the wayside in having a mistress and fathering a bastard. Descartes replied that human foibles should be treated with charity and understanding, and that no one living should disdain the mundane pleasures of love.

I know you might think Descartes was a conservative. But while he wore the conventional green velvet and a wig, he was also working night and day to replace Aristotle with Cartesian physics and St. Thomas Aquinas with Cartesian theology. He was one of those philosophers whose faith in reason was so strong that he thought that by writing a book he could change the world.